Medical Astrology for Healing

Thaya Edwards

General Disclaimer: This book is provided for information purposes only, with no guarantee of accuracy; it is not intended as a substitute for medical advice, nor as a claim for its effectiveness in treating any symptoms or disease. If symptoms persist, seek professional medical advice; minor symptoms can often be a sign of a more serious underlying condition.

The American Federation of Asrologers does not accept any responsibility for the consequences of any action taken as a result of any of the content of this book, and makes no warranties regarding the value or utility of the information and resources contained in this book.

Copyright 2015 by Thaya Edwards

No part of this book may be reproduced or transcribed in any form or by any means, electronic or mechanical, including photocopying or recording or by any information storage and retrieval system without written permission from the author and publisher, except in the case of brief quotations embodied in critical reviews and articles. Requests and inquiries may be mailed to: American Federation of Astrologers, Inc., 6535 S. Rural Road, Tempe, AZ 85283.

ISBN-10: 0-86690-659-2
ISBN-13: 978-0-86690-659-3

Cover Design: Jack Cipolla

Published by:
American Federation of Astrologers, Inc.
6535 S. Rural Road
Tempe, AZ 85283

www.astrologers.com

Contents

Preface	v
Introduction	vii
Chapter 1, Astroanatomy and Astrophysiology	1
Chapter 2, Metabolism of Zodiac Signs	11
Chapter 3, Aspects in Medical Astrology	19
Chapter 4, The Medical Horoscope	23
Chapter 5, Degrees	31
Chapter 6, Fixed Stars in Medical Astrology	39
Chapter 7, The Hyleg and the Antihyleg	43
Chapter 8, Astrodiagnosis	55
Chapter 9, How to Read a Medical Chart	63
Chapter 10, Prediction of Time when Illness Might Occur	71
Chapter 11, The Horoscope of Disease	89
Chapter 12, Lunar Days	93
Chapter 13, The Moon in the Signs: Choosing the Time for Surgery and Much More	101
Chapter 14, How to Use Medical Astrology in Healing Practice	105
Medical Glossary	121
Appendix 1. Ephemeris of Proserpina	125
Appendix 2. Decans, Terms and Degree Rulers in a Medical Chart	141
Appendix 3. Planetary Hours	143
Bibliography	145

Preface

When I asked a few well-known North American astrologers to read my manuscript and give me their honest opinion, all three of them spoke in unison: yes, this is impressive, a huge amount of work, but. . . . "But" meant that the book is a bit controversial: a lot of the information presented here is as yet unknown in North America. Where did you get this information? Bibliography please!

All my information comes from Russia. When I started to study astrology in the early 1980s, there were no astrological books available in Russia. Even the Sun-sign horoscopes so common in North American newspapers were forbidden. Our teacher, Pavel Globa, was extremely knowledgeable, although we didn't know how or where he managed to accumulate this knowledge. He was an historian and we, his students of astrology, speculated that he may have had access to some closed archives and that perhaps his grandfather had taught him (there were astrologers in pre-communist Russia).

All that we, the students of such underground groups, had were our notes and our determination. Russia itself is between the West and the East, and our astrological school (which later became known as the Avestal School of Astrology) combined Hellenistic, Indian, ancient Arabian, and modern astrology. Some astrologers might disagree with this "medley," but I just love it. Even if I didn't accept some fictitious planets that Pavel Globa introduced later, from my own experience I could see that Proserpina and the Black and White Moons work.

The only other book about medical astrology we could get in Russia was Raphael's (as an underground photocopy, of course). Unfortunately, it could not add anything to what I had already learned. I have never stopped learning and seeking information, but rarely do I find something to add to the knowledge I received thirty years ago in a country where the practice of astrology was forbidden.

When I moved to Canada, in 2003, I was surprised to find almost no books about medical astrology, and that astrology itself is much less understood and respected than it is in modern Russia. What I hope to accomplish through this book is to share my knowledge and experience. I am generally a very practical person and, being an energy healer as well, I would like to see the results of my learning and practice passed along to others. After all, that's how I know that this system works.

Best wishes,
Thaya Edwards

Introduction

This book is in many ways different from other books on the same subject. It is more practical than theoretical and includes information about which many North American astrologers are unfamiliar.

I am originally from Russia, where astrology has finally become a respected science. It wasn't like that when I first began practicing astrology in communist Russia in the early 1980s. At that time astrology was banned, along with many other things (yoga, karate, tai-chi, esoteric and religious practices, rock and roll, Coca-Cola, and other things from the West), and we were forced to study in underground groups, the farther from the all-seeing eyes of the KGB the better. In 2003, I moved to Canada, where I continued practicing and teaching astrology.

My interest in medical astrology stems from the fact that I'm also an energy healer and, in addition, work with herbs and aromatherapy. In my youth I received training as a military nurse, which helped me to better understand how a human body works.

This book is intended for two kinds of readers: astrologers and healers. In principle, this book can be read by anyone; however, in order to understand it one should have a basic knowledge of astrology. I assume the reader already understands the basics and therefore don't discuss them here.

There is a lot of information in this book that you can't find in other sources. The description of the planets, signs, and houses from a medical point of view is probably the same. However, I use a different house system based on the moments of sunrise and sunset, as well as a couple of additional planets (Proserpina, for example). The lists of degrees and fixed stars and nebulas that have an influence on health conditions are presented in the book. Formulas for calculating Arabian Parts (Pars of Health and Pars of Disease) are also here.

Having established this basis, we then learn how to diagnose possible illnesses. My approach may seem unusual or complex, but health matters are not simple matters. In order to avoid adding to patients' problems we must be absolutely certain in what we do. This takes time and knowledge.

The possible time of disease occurrence is also considered in this book. To illustrate, the charts of my patients are used (their names are omitted for the sake of confidentiality), along with the charts of certain famous people. You will also find unique and helpful information about lunar days (information not known in North America).

In the last chapter we address the main goal of this book, the very reason it was written: in order to heal more effectively, or better yet to prevent disease altogether, one must know in advance the body's weak spots, the good and bad planets, and so on. This is where I see a big help for healers.

It is extremely important to know the most positive planet in a medical chart—the Hyleg—and the most evil—the Antihyleg. Influencing the organ or the chakra connected to the Hyleg planet, the healer can energize the patient most effectively and aid recovery. It is also useful to know the influence of lunar phases and lunar days.

Physicians of ancient times always consulted the planets, and particularly the Moon, when healing their patients. Those that practiced astrology had a high recovery rate (and that's before antibiotics were even discovered). They always paid attention to the transit of the Moon through the signs when performing surgery. All this knowledge has been undeservedly forgotten by many. Contraindications for surgery connected with the position of the Moon will clearly invoke the most criticism from traditional medicine, certain in its infallibility. However, it would be shameful not to use ancient knowledge if it lowers the risk of accidents and complications during surgery. This information can be found in this book.

There is also a large section dedicated to herbs and the time of their gathering and use. This is a science of its own. Applying certain methods, one could prevent future illnesses. I tested these methods in practice. Actually, I test everything in practice; only after I verify that the method works can I be sure of it. There are a small number of strictly theoretical chapters in my book, as they might be helpful. If there are practices I do not use, I openly mention this. But you can still try them, in case they work for you.

As for the herbs, I have vast experience in collecting them and preparing them in the appropriate hour, in accordance with the Elven (Fairy) Star (or the Chaldean row). The calculation of hours may seem difficult and painstaking (if you don't have proper software), but it will pay off, as it considerably increases the effectiveness of healing. Herbalists and energy healers may find chapter fourteen especially helpful.

I hope this book will bring you perceptible benefits and will allow us to return to the natural methods from which we have so unwisely distanced ourselves.

Sincerely,
Thaya Edwards

Chapter One

Astroanatomy and Astrophysiology

Connection Between the Human Body and the Four Fundamental Elements

Since the human body is an inherently balanced and closed system, it carries a demonstration of all four natural elements: fire, water, earth, and air. As a reminder, fire and air are active male (yang) elements, and earth and water are passive female (yin) ones.

The fire element is the main carrier of life energy, or "prana." Fire, in particular, makes a person active and energetic. With a lack of this element a person becomes apathetic and weak, whereas an excess of it also would not be good (especially with the afflicted planets in fire signs). An excess of non-sublimated energy can lead to tumors or the destruction of cells.

The earth element is associated with dense body tissues such as bones and cartilage. In afflicted earth signs there appears a tendency to the formation of stones, salt deposition, and hypertrophied bone growth.

The air element relates to links within the body. It is in charge of the breathing process and is responsible for nerve fibers and all of the connective tissues.

The water element is associated with all fluids inside the body: blood, lymph, gastric juices, urine, interstitial fluid, and bile. The endocrine system also applies to the water element. Water is the most precarious element, responding to external stimuli just as well as to psychological instability.

Each of the four elements has its principal organ—which appears to be its energy center—in the human body. The ancients considered these organs as sacred, believing that they held spirits of the elements. Through these organs it is possible to balance the elements, if you know their active hours and the appropriate techniques.

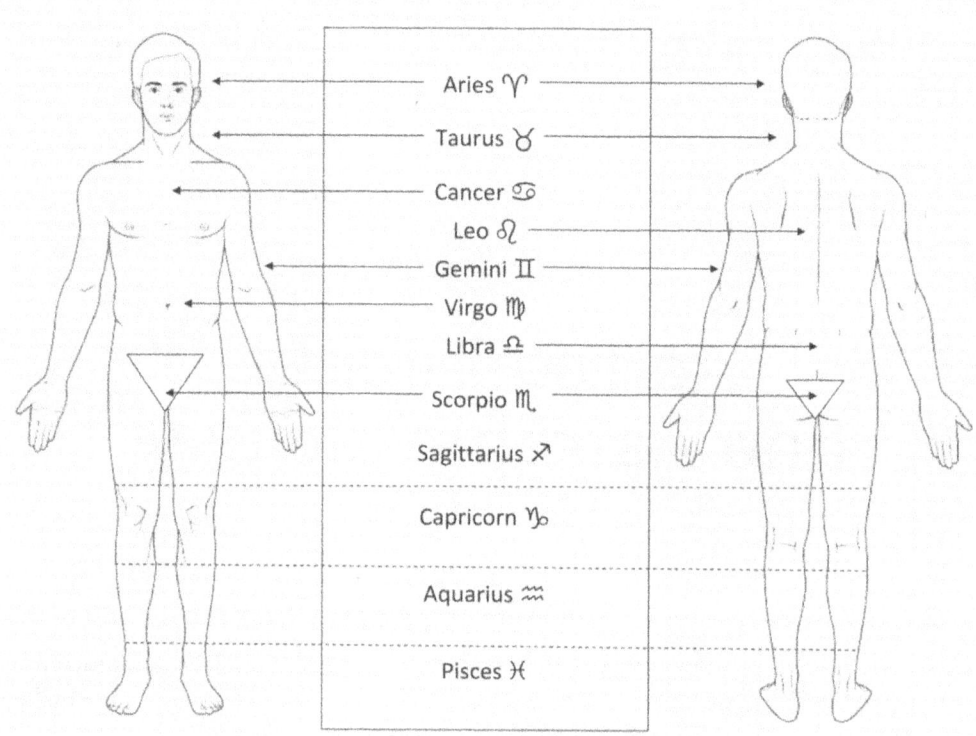

Figure 1. Zodiac and the Human Body

The fire element has its own energy center in the *heart*, the keeper of life and creative enthusiasm. For earth, it is the *sexual organs*: the ovaries for women and the prostate for men; the organs of reproduction. The air element is associated with the *lungs*, which provide a connection with the surrounding space. The sacred organ of the water element is the *liver*, our alchemical lab, which serves many functions: cleaning, assimilation, conversion, and haemopoiesis (formation of blood cellular components).

Strengthening one or another element may be possible by influencing its principal organ at a certain time of a day. Working with the fire element should be done from sunrise to noon; with water, from noon until sunset; air, from sunset until midnight; and earth, from midnight to sunrise.

Connection Between Elements and Diseases

Fire diseases. In general, these illnesses occur because of overstrain and overwork—physical as well as mental. Physical illnesses are associated with a violation of thermal exchange, and include fever and inflammation as well as heart, liver and head diseases. These diseases usually take an acute course, sometimes with mobility impairments. Mental illnesses of the Fire element include unmotivated irritability, short temper and aggressiveness.

Earth diseases are associated with a lack of heat, hypothermia and the deposition of salts, as well as sand and stones in the kidneys, gallbladder and bladder, arthritis and degenerative discs disease. Mental earth illnesses are depression, withdrawal and hypochondria. Diseases of the earth element usually have a protracted, chronic form.

People with a horoscope of fire, earth, or fire-earth are less prone to acquired diseases because they are less susceptible to external influences, including epidemics. More often they have inherited or karmic diseases.

Air illnesses are respiratory diseases, dysfunction of the autonomic nervous system, hypertension, hypotension, dermatitis (as an effect of skin allergies), neuritis, neuralgia, and convulsions. Mental illnesses are neurosis and a manic-paranoid syndrome. Air element diseases often have vague symptoms.

Water diseases are blood and lymph ailments, edemas, and dropsy. Mental illnesses are delirium, depression, and manias. Here, too, we find drug addiction, including alcoholism. Water diseases are protracted, sluggish.

People with a horoscope of air, water, or water-air have a tendency to acquired diseases, received from contact with other people.

Zodiac Reflection on the Human Body

Being a miniature "outer space," we have reflections of all twelve zodiac signs in our body (Figure 1). Organs are also associated with signs and, more specifically, with planets. We must bear in mind that two or three planets could be responsible for some organs. Let's examine the correspondence of signs and human body parts.

Aries: head (without the lower jaw), face.

Taurus: lower jaw, neck, thyroid and parathyroid glands, tonsils, adenoids, vocal cords, upper part of the esophagus.

Gemini: shoulders, arms and wrists, collarbone, thymus gland, trachea, bronchi and lungs.

Cancer: chest, breast, stomach, diaphragm.

Leo: back (from neck to waist), upper part of backbone, heart.

Virgo: intestine (without the rectum), peritoneum, upper abdomen, solar plexus.

Libra: small of the back, top of the pelvis, kidneys, bladder, skin.

Scorpio: lower abdomen, rectum, genitals, bones of the nose.

Sagittarius: buttocks, lower part of the pelvis, thighs, hips, sciatic nerve. Also related to the liver through Jupiter.

Capricorn: knees and gallbladder.

Aquarius: shins to ankle joints, blood circulation, autonomic nervous system.

Pisces: feet and ankles, lymphatic system.

Precise knowledge of divisions of the human body according to zodiac signs is a necessary attribute for determining the appropriate timing for surgery.

Planets and the Senses

Three planets control *vision*: the Sun, the Moon, and Mercury.

Hearing is controlled by Saturn. Afflicted Saturn sometimes gives deafness, especially if it is in the twelfth house close to the Ascendant. If Saturn is eastern (i.e. located to the east of the Sun), the right ear is more affected; if it is western, then the left one will suffer the most.

Venus is responsible for *touch*, Mars for *taste*, and Jupiter for *smell*.

If these planets are affected by negative aspects, malfunctions of the senses can be observed.

Planets and Function of Tissues

The **Sun** generates smooth muscles tissue, which is not controlled by our will (muscles of the heart, stomach, etc.). The Sun is not subject to control in a chart because it is a reflection of our consciousness.

The **Moon** is responsible for body fluids (lymph, blood plasma).

Mercury forms connective tissue (ligaments, tendons).

Venus is related to adipose tissue.

Mars is responsible for the striated muscles, which are controlled by our will. If Mars is strong there are well-developed muscles; if Mars is weak the muscles can be flabby, underdeveloped.

Jupiter forms skin tissue, the epithelium.

Saturn is related to bones, including teeth.

Uranus governs the nervous tissue.

Neptune forms glandular tissues (all glands of internal secretion).

Pluto is connected to all tumors and scar tissue.

Proserpina forms hair, nails, eyebrows and eyelashes (Proserpina is an unknown planet in Western astrology. See the explanation below.).

Chiron is associated with blood and lymph.

Planets and the Organs They Control

The human body has an imprint of the twelve zodiacal signs, and each organ has a planetary ruler. Particularly important are the organs controlled by the seven visible planets.

The **Sun** is associated with the **heart** and the big circle of blood circulation and is a supplier of energy.

The **Moon** controls the **stomach** and gastrointestinal tract and is responsible for the assimilation and transformation of substances.

Mercury is associated with the **lungs**, respiratory system and vocal cords. Together with the Moon, Mercury is related to the autonomic nervous system and all functions connected to it.

Venus controls the **kidneys** and urinary system as a whole. It is related to the endocrine system, especially the thyroid gland.

Mars is associated with the **brain** and is responsible for the level of iron in the blood.

Jupiter governs the **liver** and the small circle of blood circulation. The liver is the alchemical laboratory of the body.

Saturn is associated with the **spinal cord**, as well as the gall bladder and pancreas. It is directly responsible for the hematopoietic function of the spinal cord. Saturn also governs bones and teeth.

Ancient physicians used only the above seven planets. The rest of the planets, starting with Uranus, came into use later as they were discovered. However, it is known that many physicians and alchemists of the East more than a thousand years ago knew of the existence of farther planets even though they could not see them. They even knew about the existence of Proserpina, which has not yet been discovered. Nowadays we cannot ignore the planets of the higher octave, as they play an increasingly important role in our lives, including our health.

Uranus is related to the **cerebellum**. It is also relevant to the vascular system; for example, changes in blood pressure are directly related to Uranus. Uranus is also a center of orientation in time and space. It is sort of a biological clock in the body.

Neptune is associated with the **pancreas** and its many functions in the regulation of metabolism. It refers to all endocrine glands and the nervous system as a whole.

Pluto relates to the **genitals**.

Proserpina controls the **immune system** and regeneration. It is also associated with the spleen.

Chiron controls **homeostasis**.

Proserpina and Chiron are lesser-known planets, and Proserpina is generally unknown in Western astrology. Therefore, I will give more information on these two.

Proserpina

Proserpina is an as yet undiscovered planet located beyond Pluto. She is very slow; her cycle is about 665 years. Proserpina transits one degree in two years. (An ephemeris of Proserpina can be found in Appendix 1.)

Proserpina was first introduced by Russian astrologer Pavel Globa, who apparently took the concept from ancient East-Indian astrology. For some reason Indian astrologers knew about Proserpina and other farther planets long ago, even without modern technology.

I always check to see if any new information regarding astrology works for me. Proserpina always works in my astrological and healing practices—especially in medical astrology—which is why I didn't question its existence when, upon moving to Canada, I discovered that few North American astrologers used it.

Proserpina is responsible for the transformation and irreversible changes in our lives. She is the main planet of medicine, chemistry and alchemy.

Proserpina is a planet of the earth element and Yin energy. Her home is in Virgo (along with Mercury), exaltation in Gemini, detriment in Pisces, and fall in Sagittarius. Due to the fact that this planet is very slow, Proserpina plays an important role only in horoscopes where she is located in a special position, such as conjunction the Ascendant or Midheaven. She is always visible in transits, for which the acceptable orb is eighteen minutes; even with this orb the transit lasts about six months. Because this is a book on medical astrology, I'm not going to discuss here how the transits of Proserpina affect events in our lives (but believe me, there are a lot of exciting things to say).

In medicine Proserpina is associated with the immune system as well as growth of hair, nails, eyebrows, and eyelashes. As the planet of transformation, the role of Proserpina in the process of regeneration of damaged tissues is extremely high. A few people with a strong and kind Proserpina located at the angular points of the chart have a phenomenal ability to survive in extreme situations and to regenerate tissues. It is believed that they were even able to force their mental will to engage the recovery of damaged organs in their original form. As fantastic as it may sound, the process of full recovery is not impossible. If the lizard can grow a new tail, why cannot people regenerate damaged or missing body parts?

Proserpina is associated with near-death experiences and the return to life. She also has a connection to some sexually transmitted diseases. For example, it is believed that she is involved in the formation of AIDS because its appearance coincided with Proserpina's entrance to Scorpio (this sign is directly related to sexually transmitted diseases). Well, you might disagree with this concept because Pluto moved to Scorpio almost at the same time. And you may be right. Anyway, the fact that two of them happened to be in Scorpio definitely made matters worse. Proserpina has a relation to any kind of mutation and sometimes is involved in the occurrence of cancer (examples in following chapters).

Chiron

Chiron is a planet recognized by many astrologers, but the approach to it is different in various astrological schools. In fact, Chiron was originally considered to be an asteroid with an odd trajectory and a cycle of 50.78 years. Since then astronomers have concluded that Chiron represents an unusually large comet nucleus and it is classified as a minor planet.

In the majority of astrological schools, Chiron, as "a wounded healer," is related to our deepest spiritual wounds and our ability to heal them.

In the Avestan School of Astrology (where I studied), Chiron is considered a planet of balance, harmony and justice; a mediator. Chiron is a planet of the air element, Den (neutral) energy. His home is in Libra (with Venus), exaltation in Sagittarius, detriment in Aries, and fall in Gemini.

In medical astrology Chiron does not mean much and is poorly studied. His main function is to maintain homeostasis (balance) of the organism. It is also believed that he is connected with the endocrine system via the adrenal glands; he has influence on the immune system, hormone production, and lymph circulation. It is noticed that a person with a strong and kind Chiron won't be affected by radiation.

In my opinion, it makes sense to pay attention to Chiron in a medical chart only if he is located at the angular points or in the sixth or twelfth houses. Location of Chiron in these houses brings difficulties in diagnostics and changeable courses of illnesses. The same applies if, at the beginning of the illness, transiting Chiron was in the negative aspects: it imparts a fickle course to the disease, vague symptoms, fever, and over-excitation. If Chiron is in conjunction with any other planet and there are bad aspects involved, we can say that the disease of the planet in conjunction with Chiron will be very difficult to diagnose. Also it is likely that this disease will transfer to other organs and can disturb the equilibrium of the whole organism.

It is believed (according to the Avestan Astrological School) that Chiron will soon lose its significance and will be replaced with another as yet undiscovered planet, Vulcan. Vulcan is located between Mercury and the Sun, making it the closest planet to the Sun. This is a planet of cosmic laws and connection to higher intelligence. For now it is in a hidden state, and I have never seen any signs of Vulcan's influence.

Lilith and Lunar Nodes in a Medical Chart

Lilith, or the Black Moon, is a fictional planet and in medical astrology is not always taken into account. However, the influence of Lilith can be huge if it was in a prominent position at the beginning of an illness, in which case it always aggravates the disease. Depending on its position in the horoscope and the aspects, Lilith may have a different effect.

First, the Black Moon indicates a shift of the disease onto the mentality, to the extent of the emergence of psychosis and suicide attempts on the grounds of illness. Second, the location of Lilith in the fourth house indicates the likelihood of genetic diseases, often associated with a hereditary curse. Official medicine does not cure such diseases. Third, Lilith is also associated with illnesses not indicated in the natal chart, but provoked by black magic. These diseases are of artificial origin and are associated with negative energy impacts, consisting of the "evil eye," curses, energy vampirism, etc. Such diseases are treated exclusively by special methods.

The lunar nodes do not have a particular value in a medical horoscope by themselves; only their aspects are considered. Conjunction of a North Node with a planet indicates diseases of this planet with a Jupiter tint (i.e. systemic form), and the conjunction of a South Node provides a Saturn tint (chronic form). Negative aspects of the lunar nodes could also be indicators of karmic diseases that cannot be cured without their elaboration on the inner spiritual level.

Planets and Specific Diseases

The **Sun** is associated with blood circulation disorders, heart disorders (including heart attacks), and fainting. Negative aspects of the Sun and Moon give visual impairment and eye diseases.

The **Moon** is associated with neurological disorders, diseases of the stomach and its mucous membrane, and a violation of gastric acidity. Accumulation of fluid in tissues can also be referred to the Moon.

Mercury is associated with respiratory diseases (catarrh, bronchitis, pneumonia), and with speech *disorders* (e.g. stuttering).

Venus is associated with kidney illnesses and urinary tract infections (cystitis, nephritis, etc.).

Mars is responsible for various erysipelatous diseases, acne, hemorrhoids, abscesses, open sores and meningitis.

Jupiter is associated with liver (hepatitis, cholecystitis, etc.) and lung (pneumonia, pleurisy) ailments.

Saturn is associated with stones in the kidneys and gallbladder, diseases of salt exchange (arthritis, rheumatism, sciatica, osteochondrosis), and tooth decay.

Uranus is associated with neuroses, stroke, hypo- and hypertension.

Neptune is associated with various mental illnesses, alcoholism, and drug addiction. It can produce a comatose state, as well as poisoning by medications. When Neptune is afflicted all medicine should be taken very carefully lest it lead to intoxication.

Pluto is associated with cancer.

Proserpina is associated with immune system disorders.

For complex diseases, for which several planets are responsible, other rules apply. We will get into details about them in following chapters.

Planets and Clinical Courses

Different people are affected by illness in different ways. Some have acute illnesses with fevers and crises consuming a lot of strength, but with rapid recovery after the crisis. Other diseases are sluggish and lingering, often moving into a chronic stage, with a slow recovery. Such diseases can exhaust a person more than illnesses of a crisis character. The ailing person is not going to die, but does not have a normal life.

The specificity of the course of a disease is also determined by planets. Which course of a disease a person will be most inclined to shows in a sign of the sixth house and the planets in it.

The **Sun** and **Moon** have no role in the formation of the disease, but other planets of a classical group can provide the necessary information.

Mars can be seen immediately in the course of the disease. Illnesses are sudden and acute with inflammations and fevers.

Saturn appears as a lasting chronic disease with recurring symptoms.

Mercury gives unstable chronic diseases and changeable course of the illness with sudden exacerbations.

Jupiter is associated with a systemic form of diseases, in which the overall system of organs is affected (e.g. the endocrine system).

Venus is responsible for latent (hidden) forms of the illness.

Any illness may begin in a latent form, and then transform into another. Often the acute Mars form of a disease can transform into a lasting chronic form of Saturn or an unstable chronic form of Mercury. All these transformations can be tracked in a horoscope by paying attention to transits and some other indicators.

Chapter Two

Metabolism of the Signs

In this chapter we'll look at the metabolism of different signs and also the main recommendations about proper diet, lifestyle, etc. Besides that we will see how people with the different signs behave when they are ill.

These of course are just general concepts. Astrology is an exact science. It is pointless to divide mankind into twelve groups and give everyone the same recommendations in any sphere. General conclusions work only for typical representatives of signs which make up just one third of the populace. If there is a stellium (a group of planets) in the sign different from the Sun sign, we can talk about an atypical sign's representative. Such a person most likely will manifest more of the stellium sign than the Sun sign.

When we talk about illnesses related to the signs, this is just predisposition. Illness might not happen if planets in the sign are not afflicted. It is necessary to have at least two levels of affliction for disease to develop. Levels of affliction might include a planet participating in the Grand Cross or T-square patterns or a planet in its fall or detriment, in a negative critical degree (see Chapter Five), or as an Anti-Hyleg (see Chapter Seven) etc.

Aries

Aries individuals have a fast metabolism so their illnesses are usually acute, fast and sudden, with a high fever and with recovery following a crisis.

A gathering of afflicted planets in Aries may lead to nervous over-fatigue, nervous breakdown, and insomnia. Aries individuals have weak blood vessels with a tendency to spasms (stroke can't be excluded), which is why they should not smoke and should avoid everything that could provoke vessel spasms. In cold weather they should cover their heads. There is a possibility of frequent migraines because of vessel spasms.

Because Saturn is in its fall in Aries, problems with the bone system are possible (especially with teeth). Dental problems bring big stress in the life of Aries individuals, and despite their bravery they are terribly afraid of pain, especially toothache. Visiting a dentist is, for them, an exploit more frightening than walking on a rope over an abyss. If someone faints while at the dentist, it is most likely an Aries.

Aries individuals can have a so-called nervous fever, when after feeling nervous they have a suddenly high temperature, but they are not sick. Kids may have cramps in addition to fever, even seizures looking like epilepsy. However, it generally isn't epilepsy; it is just functional convulsions because of a compromised metabolism.

Aries individuals are difficult patients. He or she can't stay in bed, gets nervous because of being idle, and is always ready to run somewhere.

For good metabolism Aries individuals should take enough potassium and iron with food (better with veggies and fruits), and lots of protein for the proper functioning of muscles. I have no intention of being a substitute for a nutritionist here, but I will list some products containing the mentioned micro-elements.

For example, sources of potassium are apricots, broccoli, orange juice, bananas, soy beans, avocado, pomegranates, turnip, and meat. Meat (mostly beef) is the best source of iron. Aries are rarely vegetarians, but for those who are, here are more foods containing iron: beans, lentils, peas, lettuce, spinach, tofu, unpeeled potatoes, whole-wheat bread, starch, and molasses.

I also offer a couple more pieces of advice about preventive measures and keeping oneself healthy. First of all, Aries individuals need to know how to relax and reduce the tension put on the nervous system. It is important to have enough sleep. From time to time they should take several days of complete rest from all concerns. They should control aggressiveness that might do harm to themselves and the people around them.

Taurus

This earth sign is associated with a somewhat slow metabolism, which is why food, when there is too much of it, easily turns into fat. Taurus' like to eat well. When they are hungry, this immediately affects their mood: they become discontented, irritated, and even angry. Parents should be careful in feeding their Taurus kids: for them it's better to be skinny than plump because if cells get used to having lots of food, later it will be very difficult to change (cells will demand more and more food).

Food should contain a lot of vitamins A and E, and enough iodine. The main source of iodine is seafood (laminaria especially). Iodized salt would also help. The product containing the biggest amount of vitamin A is liver (especially beef liver). Vitamin A is also found in carrots, tomatoes, eggs, and milk and other dairy products. For vitamin E we will need soy oil as well as sunflower oil, dairy products, soy beans, liver, flower, carrots, tomatoes, and bananas.

Weak parts of the body for Taurus are the throat and thyroid gland. There also might be sinus problems. Because of their slow metabolism, Taurus could have skin problems such as a dry, allergic rash. Elder Taurus individuals (if the sign is afflicted) also have a tendency to heart attack, diabetes, hepatitis, and joint diseases.

A sick Taurus recovers very slowly; illnesses linger and often turn chronic. Taurus individuals originally have good regeneration, but it tends to slow down.

The main prophylaxis for Taurus: don't overeat, watch the amount of drinking, and take care of nasopharynx (sinus, in simple words). Different kinds of immunity stimulation are good for Taurus (even polar bear swims).

Gemini

Gemini's metabolism is very fast—so fast that it might cause a lack of oxygen in blood. Oxygen is used up quickly and toxins aren't eliminated from the body fast enough, resulting in their circulating in the blood for a long time. This might result in skin problems (rash, acne, and so on). Originally, Geminis have good immunity, but their wounds don't heal fast. Geminis have a somewhat weak nervous system. They are very mobile, have lots of interests and want to be in several places simultaneously which might lead to nervous exhaustion. There is a possibility of respiratory diseases, problems with arms and speech disorders if the sign of Gemini is afflicted.

Geminis often try to find non-existent ailments in themselves. We can diagnose "chronic hypochondria" for this sign. By the way, they can have any kind of disease because of their nerves, so if a Gemini gets stressed out, he or she may feel a pain in any organ: liver, heart, etc. It is clear psychosomatics.

Geminis don't like having medical treatment. They tend to try different kinds of medications, but don't have the patience to finish a course of treatment and are likely to just give up. They also trust commercials: drugs that are on the screen are the best.

Preventive measures for them include spending more time in fresh air, strengthening their respiratory system (maybe using breathing practices), getting enough sleep, not smoking, and controlling their emotions. For good metabolism they need enough phosphorus and calcium with their food. Microelement phosphorus is contained in nuts (cashews, almonds), beans, chocolate, mushrooms, milk and dairy products, meat, and fish. As for calcium, it is in dairy products, laminaria (kelp), nuts, molasses, beans, oranges, broccoli, rutabaga, sardines, and soy milk. Vitamin D is needed for calcium assimilation.

Cancer

Their metabolism depends a lot on the condition of their liquids. The most vulnerable parts for Cancers are the lymphatic and urinary systems. If there is something wrong with their metabolism, they may have edemas, dropsy, weeping dermatitis, or ailments of the urinary tract. Cancers are well known for their high emotional excitability. They may have psychosomatic disorders that hide the real disease, which is why sometimes they receive incorrect treatment.

If the sign is afflicted there is a possibility of digestion disorders and diseases of the gastrointestinal tract (colitis, gastritis, etc). Cancers are very sensitive to outside factors; their original resistibility isn't good. Usually they have poor regeneration of tissues and they recover slowly after surgery and traumas.

Their diseases linger. Cancer children often have all sorts of childhood diseases (whooping cough, measles, mumps). A sick Cancer is hypochondriac; this individual can actually create a disease if he or she thinks often enough about it, even though it hasn't occurred naturally. Cancers can hardly bear pain. Treatments that affect the electrical condition of body liquids are positive for Cancers; this can include physiotherapy or energy healing.

For good metabolism they should have enough calcium and fluorine with their food. Food products containing calcium were mentioned above. Fluorine can be found in fish, whole wheat, tea, eggs, and liver.

For preventive measures for Cancers it is good to strengthen the nervous system and be more active (walking, hiking, etc.) with the purpose of improving the circulation of fluids. They shouldn't sleep too much during a Full Moon and food shouldn't be heavy. Cancers need to take care of the work of the alimentary tract.

Leo

For typical Leos the weakest organ is the heart. Leos often overstrain because they overestimate their energy. As a result they may have functional neurosis, including neurosis of the heart. Their metabolism depends in some way on nerve conduction (through nerve fibers). Lots of stress impairs nerve conduction, and that in turn affects the heart rate. Leos might even have a fibrillation, making it impossible to count how many heartbeats they have in a minute.

In the case of an afflicted sign there might be such illnesses as angina, aortic dissection, hypertension, heart attack, and illnesses of the upper thoracic area of the backbone.

Sometimes Leos have a low level of albumen in their blood plasma. Leos are very sensitive to radiation, even to the sun's radiation, although they have a good immune system and their illnesses are acute with fast recovery.

A sick Leo doesn't look sick and always says that he or she is okay. They don't want to stay in bed. Care should be taken with these patients as their health condition can be underestimated. In diagnosing, there always needs to be a heart control. Leos have a good reaction to naturopathy, including herbs, honey, and so on.

Leos need food with a lot of protein to support the albumen level of their blood plasma, and less sugar and starch. The main microelement they need is magnesium. Magnesium is contained in tea, dairy products, cereals, cacao beans, and some other products in very small amounts. The most useful vitamins are C and E. Vitamin E was mentioned already. Vitamin C can be found in all fruits and veggies, especially in citrus plants. Rosehips (wild rose) are the richest source of vitamin C.

For preventive measures Leos should spend more time with nature, training their heart and blood vessels, and doing exercises for the spine, and limit their time in the sun.

Virgo

The affliction of a Virgo sign almost always brings disorders in the workings of the intestines. Nervous overload can also lead to digestion disorders, and Virgo children often experience diarrhea. Virgo's metabolism fully depends on the condition of intestines. Virgos should be especially careful in the matter of nutrition. It is helpful for them to do some form of purification from time to time, and they should take care of their nervous system.

A patient of this sign is a difficult one for a doctor or a healer, because he or she is very suspicious and pays a great deal of attention to small details. Usually they don't like to take medications. Their ailments are difficult to diagnose: they have latent symptoms that develop very slowly.

Virgos should avoid spicy food and products that are hard to digest. Their food should be rich with protein. The most important mineral is potassium.

The main part of preventive measures is their diet. And of course Virgos should avoid stress because stress affects the intestines and the state of the intestines affects their metabolism.

Libra

Libra's metabolism is fast, unstable, and sensitive to influences from external factors. The immune system is also unstable and easily worsens with stress. With the sign's affliction the main illness is disease of the kidneys and urinary tract. Secretion system dysfunctions may cause a high level of toxins which in turn lead to skin ailments such as dermatitis, allergy rash, or dry skin. Kidney dysfunction is often accompanied by high blood pressure and headaches. Libras also can suffer from radiculitis and sciatica.

Consuming too many sweets can be dangerous and it would be worthwhile to check blood sugar levels from time to time. Libras need phosphorus and sodium for good metabolism, though the amount of sodium should be balanced: too much or too little isn't good. Sodium chloride is in common table salt and sodium is also found in goat milk and celery. Sodium plays a huge role in the body's water-salt balance.

Sick Libras love receiving lots of attention and care, which is why they sometimes are inclined to simulation: to recover later and get more attention. Because Libras are sensitive, their family doctor should be nice and patient. Their family should create a good, cheerful atmosphere at home for sick Libras; otherwise patients would stay in bed for a long time.

Libras should strenghten their nervous system as a preventive measure. Meditation and self-hypnosis are helpful for this. They need enough physical exercise, especially for the spine. Libras should always watch the condition of their kidneys and blood sugar levels.

Scorpio

Scorpio's metabolism is fast, and because this is a water sign it depends on a physicochemical structure of liquids in the body. This structure in turn depends on the fluctuation of the magnetic field and other geophysical factors, to which Scorpios are very sensitive. They can be prone to poisoning. The cells' metabolism is the most vulnerable. With an afflicted sign there is a possibility of ailments of the rectum (piles) and genitals. This sign also has a tendency to the formation of tumors. There is a danger of venereal diseases (if one creates conditions for this, of course).

Diet should include vitamins B, C, E, and plenty of iron, calcium, and protein.

A sick Scorpio is very patient, doesn't like to complain, and usually doesn't pay attention to sickness, which is why they often miss the early stages of disease (when it is easier to cure). If a Scorpio begins to complain it means that things are really bad. Scorpios usually don't trust doctors, but they are very active in struggling with illnesses if they decide to take treatments.

Their infections and inflammations are acute, but fortunately Scorpios are tough, have good survival skills, and recover fairly rapidly.

The preventive measure for them is temperance in everything—in food, drink, and sex. And of course a balanced diet with all necessary nutrients is helpful.

Sagittarius

Sagittarius' metabolism is active and fast and depends on the state of the nervous system and the production of detoxifying agents: antibodies, leucocytes, phagocytes, and ferments. These people should avoid overeating because of possible overloading for the liver. Their nervous system needs good care because any ailment can become acute if they are stressed out. They suffer from overstrain a lot if they work for too long a time without good rest.

Those with this sign are difficult to diagnose. They may have strange fevers that disappear fast but then return. Their illnesses often start with a high fever, followed by fatigue. With the sign's affliction there is a possibility of autonomic nervous system disorders, cricks, joints dislocations, sciatica, rheumatism, liver illnesses, and inner bleeding.

The Sagittarius diet should have lots of vitamins B and C, and an important mineral for them is silicon. With proper nutrition they should consume 1-3 grams of silicon daily; the foods with the most silicon are broccoli and whole cereals. There should be lots of fruits, berries, and veggies in their diet.

Sagittarius individuals are usually cheerful patients; they joke about their diseases and don't like to stay in bed. The family physician should appear reliable and follow all of the usual medical rituals; otherwise the patient will not trust the physician and will not recover. Methods of psychotherapy and naturopathic treatment work really well for Sagittarius.

As a preventive measure, Sagittarius individuals should follow a balanced lifestyle with adequate physical exercise; otherwise they will easily gain weight, especially in the hips. They shouldn't sleep in warm and stuffy rooms. It's better for them to pay attention to the first signs of pain or discomfort in the low back and hip joints because it is the way in which many of their diseases might start. It is also important to avoid stress as stress weakens their resistance.

Capricorn

Their metabolism is slow and inert, with bone tissue being the first to suffer as a result. Capricorn's digestion is usually not good and it is advisable to drink some digestive stimulants before eating. Capricorn is the only sign for which having a little bit of alcohol can be recommended. Their food should contain a lot of phosphorus and calcium (especially in winter), as well as protein and iron. Capricorns should limit fats and hot spices in their diet.

They have a good resistance to disease, but also they have an inclination to depression, which in its turn leads to poor functioning of the alimentary tract. They often have constipation and they should try to avoid this because it affects their metabolism. With the sign's affliction the typical illnesses are salt deposits, degenerative disc disease, problems with joints, and stones in the gallbladder and kidneys.

Capricorn's diseases usually linger and are not acute. They should be careful not to take too much medication. Psychotherapy is always good for them, especially when illnesses are followed by depression. A Capricorn patient is not talkative, so the doctor has to work somewhat like a veterinarian: first, identify the disease without much help from the patient, and then treat it.

Capricorn health has three main enemies: cold, moisture, and constipation, all of which should be avoided. They should also pay attention to the condition of their teeth. Exercise and massage are beneficial to Capricorn. Also they should limit salt in their diet and eat lots of vitamin-rich foods, especially in winter. The best locations for Capricorns to live in are dry highlands.

Aquarius

Aquarius metabolism might have instability because of temporary changes in blood and lymph. A lot depends on the environment. Resistance and the immune system depend on the nervous system's condition. Their sicknesses are acute and sudden, with a disorder of blood circulation in small vessels (capillaries) being common. Problems with the lymphatic system are immediately shown in blood circulation, which affects the Aquarius part of the body: lower legs. There could be varicose veins, spasms, and phlebitis.

For metabolic improvement they need food with enough phosphorus, iron, and calcium.

An Aquarius is a difficult patient. Often he or she refuses to take any treatment, instead waiting for a quick recovery by miracle. If they finally decide to go for treatment, they take the process radically. Aquarius tends to go for extreme methods without any protocol. They might switch from starvation to a nourishing diet and vice versa.

Aquarius individuals should pay attention to their blood, eyesight, and psyche, which are vulnerable when they are sick. Taking herbs is very beneficial for them. If Aquarius individuals are in good emotional shape, with an inclination to a healthy lifestyle, they will have good longevity.

Pisces

This water sign has a slow metabolism and environmental factors affect these individuals. Pisces individuals are extremely sensitive to medication, especially psychotropic drugs. Physicians should be very careful when they prescribe any kind of drug for a Pisces. These people have a weak immune system, making it necessary to use preventive measures in times of epidemics. They are also vulnerable to poisoning. Pisces has an inclination to water accumulation in tissues. There might be a disorder of the secretory function, and the nervous system is unstable.

When they are sick they can be delirious, especially if they take too much medication. Pisces individuals adapt quickly to similar kinds of drugs, so if they have a lingering disease they should change medication often. However, they must be careful to not overtake medication because their secretory function is not strong.

Pisces has an inclination to allergies, skin diseases (eczema, psoriasis), and extreme fatigue. They often feel listless and drowsy. Because of their weak immunity Pisces individuals can easily catch a cold; the respiratory system is the most vulnerable. With the sign's affliction the Pisces part of the body (feet) might suffer. They could be flat-footed, for example.

Pisces individuals can strengthen their immunity using the right diet. They need lots of sea products like laminaria and algae. Two minerals are very important: iron and sodium.

These people are easily influenced and hypochondriac. They like to read medical books, and can easily decide that they show symptoms of non-existent diseases. It is difficult to diagnose these people as they don't always identify where exactly they feel pain or discomfort; it is always in different areas. The good thing is that they take treatment seriously and have a positive reaction to almost any kind of treatment, especially physiotherapy. If you are trying to help a sick Pisces heal, recovery will be accelerated if you explain in detail what this ailment is about (such as in a medical encyclopedia) and what kind of treatment will be used. Then the patient will trust and begin to recover.

As a preventive measure, it is recommended that Pisces individuals keep their feet warm and wear comfortable shoes. Foot massage and a warm bath are good for improving blood and lymph circulation. Exercises for feet and ankle-joints are beneficial and it is good for a Pisces to ski and skate starting from early childhood.

Chapter Three

Aspects in Medical Astrology

The Main Principles of Aspect Interpretation

In this chapter we will explore two main groups of aspects: the positive and negative, as well as karmic aspects. The positive aspects are 60 degrees (sextile), 120 degrees (trine), 30 degrees (semi-sextile), and 150 degrees (quincunx) degrees; the negative are 90 degrees (square), 180 degrees (opposition), 135 degrees (sesquiquadrate), and 45 degrees (semi-square). Usually astrologers avoid referring to aspects as negative. Rather, they are called tense, challenging, or dynamic. This makes sense, as the tense aspects do not always have a negative undertone; often, they provide a stimulus for further development. However, in medical astrology, the term "negative" suits them best. It is these aspects, or more precisely three of them (90, 180, and 135 degrees), that will direct our attention when diagnosing illnesses.

Using only the aspects, without even proceeding to interpret the houses, we can determine the predisposition to certain illnesses. This is especially evident if there are tense configurations: T-square, grand cross, or pole-axe (two sesquiquadrates plus a square). For example, finding Venus in the center of a T-square, one can draw the conclusion that a person *may* experience problems with the kidneys and/or with the thyroid gland. I emphasize "may," but will it happen? We can determine this only after analyzing the entire horoscope, including the degrees, the houses, and the definition of the planetary strength and dignity. How to determine the importance and dignity of planets will be examined later with the calculation of tables of dignities.

For instance, this same Venus can have a good status in the medical horoscope. Then all the negative strength of the tense configuration will reveal itself on the level of events (problems in the love sphere, for example), and may not even affect health. Nevertheless, it is exactly the negative aspects that are the main indication of affliction.

There is another rule: it's not necessary to have aspects. An illness can manifest itself even in an empty sign if there is a gathering of planets in the opposite sign. This is because planets of the opposite sign pull the energy toward themselves, thus weakening the sign where there are no planets. Let's suppose that the sign of Taurus is empty, but that Scorpio has four or five planets. There is a strong likelihood that the person under the Taurus sign will experience problems with the neck and throat, especially in early childhood (in this case, until age fourteen). In my practice I encountered just such a case: my daughter had infantile myogenic torticollis (the head was deviated to one side), as well as constant sore throats and tonsillitis. After turning fourteen her situation improved considerably because she had entered the age of Gemini and left Taurus (here, an age progression of one sign every seven years is used).

Karmic aspects in medical astrology are little known (they are not used in Western astrology at all). In my astrological school we use four so-called karmic aspects: 20, 40, 80, and 100 degrees. In medical astrology it makes sense to pay attention to two: the novile (40 degrees) and septagon (100 degrees). They are especially indicative when working together with negative aspects. It is considered that they give the illness a protracted character and are indicators of diseases of a karmic nature, which are very difficult to treat. Illnesses of a karmic nature demand an incredible amount of patience from the afflicted person and an examination of the problem primarily on a spiritual level.

People born during an eclipse have a great chance of suffering a karmic illness. Most often, eclipses affect sensory organs, especially sight. They are also associated with incurable illnesses. However, it is important to keep in mind that not all eclipses pertain to the medical horoscope. Here again one has to look at the status of the planets. If a planet affected by an eclipse has a positive medical status, then the eclipse will not affect health. It may manifest itself only on an event level. Or, in the contrary case, it can influence only the medical, without affecting the other spheres of life.

In the first, we draw attention to tense aspects between the Sun and the Moon. Negative aspects between these two celestial bodies weaken a person's vitality. A New Moon can sometimes be considered a bad position. Children born during the New Moon are considered the weakest, especially if there are negative aspects to the New Moon. Positive aspects reduce the strength of the negative ones and give the possibility of better health.

However, it should be noted that positive stabilizing aspects do not guarantee positive results. With the strong prevalence of stabilizing aspects over the tense ones, imbalance could arise. A stabilizing aspect between two evil (according to status) planets could cause stagnant effects in the organs of the corresponding planets and signs and induce the accumulation of toxins in the body. Exactly these positive aspects, along with negative, can lead to obesity, salt deposition in the joints, arthrosclerosis, and the formation of stones.

We will discuss the aspects between the various planets in greater detail in the section "Astrodiagnostics." Now I will focus on the important topic of combust planets (a conjunction with the Sun).

Combust Planets

A planet is considered combust when it is in conjunction with the Sun within eighteen minutes to three degrees. Planets in conjunction with fewer than eighteen minutes are regarded as cazimi and will not be taken into consideration here. The Sun takes away the energy from a combust planet, with the result that the organ of this planet is weakened and an illness can occur. Combustion of a planet is not yet a diagnosis, as other indicators are required; however, this negative conjunction greatly increases the likelihood of illness. As a rule, illnesses by combust planets can be treated by energy healing through harmonizing the chakras.

Combust *Moon* brings weakness in the stomach and intestines. There will be a strong susceptibility to outside factors. This person is subject to colds and infections, and has an emotional instability which brings a series of psychosomatic illnesses. Many foods will be contra-indicated for people with a combust Moon. They need to carefully watch their diet and avoid overloading their gastro-intestinal tract.

A combust *Mercury* brings problems with speech (defects such as stuttering) if it is western (behind the Sun). If Mercury is eastern, it brings illnesses of the respiratory system.

A combust *Venus* brings illnesses of the kidneys, urinary tract, and the entire endocrine system. The metabolism of lipids can also suffer and bring about obesity.

A combust *Mars* weakens the brain and the muscular system. If Mars is western, its combustion mainly impacts the disturbance of glandular metabolism. If Mars is eastern, it brings a tendency toward brain disorders, as well as carbuncles, acne, and other skin diseases. It is very bad if the combust Mars has a square with Uranus as it strongly affects the brain's blood vessels; there might be disorders in blood circulation.

A combust *Jupiter* brings liver diseases. These people should comply with a liver-friendly diet from childhood. For example, not consuming fatty foods, as well as tomatoes and eggplant.

A combust *Saturn* can lead to disorders of the spinal function (the negative aspects of Saturn and the Sun produce the same effect). Multiple sclerosis, Bechterew's disease (Ankylosing spondylitis—see Medical Glossary), deafness, imbalance of salt metabolism, formation of stones, and diseases of the joints are also possibilities. Exposure to cold can cause the blood vessels to experience severe spasms. In this case the main preventive measure is the timely removal of toxins from the body.

A combust *Uranus* brings disorders of the autonomic nervous system, neurosis, convulsions, problems with blood vessels, and the formation of blood clots. There is also a danger of strokes and paralysis. Quite often Uranus is involved in incidences of sudden death. People with an afflicted Uranus should avoid direct sun rays and check the level of prothrombin in the blood.

A combust *Neptune* is one of the factors indicative of diabetes and blood diseases. Susceptibility to medications greatly increases and toxins remain in the blood for a long time and cause drug allergies. A significant psychological vulnerability is also noted, which can lead to mental disorders.

Alcoholism and drug addiction can't be excluded.

A combust **Pluto** can bring tissue degeneration and tumors, both benign and malignant.

A combust **Proserpina** brings disorders of biochemical processes on the cellular level (these processes are difficult to diagnose). There can also be lowered immunity and poor tissue regeneration. With the presence of a negative aspect from the combust Proserpina to the Moon, hemophilia can develop (a disease from which only men suffer and which is defined as poor clotting of the blood).

A combust Chiron brings disorders to the general homeostasis of the body.

The negative aspects of the Sun to the planets have characteristics similar to the negative conjunction (combustion).

From Simple to Complicated

As mentioned, the simple illnesses are easy to determine when one takes a look at just the aspects and planetary positions in signs. Medical houses will add much more information and make a chart more difficult to read. The significant information from houses makes diseases more complicated. Usually the illnesses revealed by aspects are simple, with clear symptoms, and they are relatively easy to treat.

For instance, a large grouping of planets afflicted by the aspects in the fire signs brings about a predisposition to the illnesses of the "fire," meaning those progressing in an acute form, with inflammations and fevers. Jupiter, when affected by negative planets, can bring about liver and gall bladder diseases, such as cholesystitis. However, it sometimes happens that Jupiter does not possess negative aspects, but a person still suffers from cholesystitis. In this case, despite similar symptoms, the illness has a different origin. Here one must consider the status of the planet Jupiter, the Parses and degrees (which will be discussed later). The same illness but with different causes should be treated in different ways.

Illnesses determined by medical houses possess a more complex character and less clear symptoms. Beginning in one area, they can spill over to another. Where, exactly, can be determined by analyzing the planet, the sign and the house in which it is located, as well as the degrees.

Now it makes sense to look at the order of the construction of a medical horoscope. The following chapter will be one of the most difficult, as it contains formulas and calculations. I urge readers to muster some patience and to refresh their mathematical knowledge.

Chapter Four

The Medical Horoscope

Construction of the Medical Horoscope

The medical system of the houses is equilateral, meaning that all the houses have the same angle of 30 degrees. The medical system I practice uses the Ascendant of Jamaspa, or Brahmagupta, named after a well-known Indian astrologer and his successor. At its foundation lies the natural cycle of the Sun with its sunrise and sunset.

This chapter will present the biggest challenges in this book. Most of us are accustomed to computers and have forgotten how to do calculations using our brain (even those who began practicing astrology before the computer era). I am going to show you a method of medical chart construction and it is up to you whether to use it or not. We will need this particular chart for figuring out Tables of Dignities and Parses (Lots) of Health and Disease.

Astrological software for the purpose of calculating medical charts does exist but is currently not available in North America. One example from Europe would be ZET, created by Anatoli Zaytsev from Ukraine (available also in English). It is possible to add new charts to the existing programs in North America and in this case my formulas will be helpful.

To find the Ascendant we need all the usual information: date, time, and place of birth. We also need the time of the sunrise and sunset for the date and place of birth. Bear in mind that leap year sunrise times may differ from those of non-leap years. Therefore, do not forget to make appropriate adjustments. The same applies to Daylight Saving Time.

The main principle of calculation is the division into night and day of the twenty-four hour period, with the assumption that half of the signs ascend during the day and half at night: 180 degrees rise during daytime and the same at night. Therefore, the speed of the ascent of one degree will be different during day and night, with the exception of an equinox. We use 360 degrees in the calculation; for example, 14 degrees of Taurus is 44 degrees (30 degrees of Aries plus 14 degrees of Taurus); 3 degrees of Sagittarius is 243 degrees; 1 degree of Aquarius is 301 degrees and so on.

From the beginning we must establish whether the person was born during the day or night. If during the day, we need the time of sunrise and sunset for that date. If at night, but before midnight, we need to find the time of sunset for the date of birth and the time of sunrise for the following date. If the birth was during night time, but after midnight, then it will be the time of sunrise on the birth date and the time of sunset on the previous date.

Let us consider an example. Suppose a person was born October 4, 2006 at 10:44 a.m. in Vancouver, Canada.

The birth occurred during the day, so we must first determine the length of the daylight hours for that day. For Vancouver, sunrise on October 4 was at 7:21 a.m., and sunset was at 6:39 p.m. (18:39 when using the 24-hour clock). To determine the length of daylight hours, we subtract 7:21 from 18:39 to get 11 hours and 18 minutes, or 678 minutes: (11 x 60) + 18 = 678.

Next we calculate the speed of ascent (V) of the zodiac sign, remembering that 180 degrees ascend during the daylight hours:

V = 678 minutes divided by 180 degrees, resulting in 3.77 minutes for each degree.

The next step is to calculate how many minutes separate the birth of the person from the time of sunrise: 10:44 – 7:21 = 3:23, which is 3 hours, 23 minutes, or 203 minutes.

Now let us find how many degrees ascended over the horizon from sunrise until the time of birth. Divide the 203 minutes between sunrise and birth by the average speed of ascent of one degree, 3.77: 203/3.77 = 53.85 degrees.

Then we need to find the Sun's coordinates at sunrise or sunset. In this case, we are looking at sunrise. At the time of sunrise, the Sun was in 11 Libra 13. To verify this, you can look up the ASC in the Placidus system. The ASC must be in the same degree. At sunrise, the Sun is positioned directly on the Ascendant. If this coordinate is converted into absolute degrees, it will become 191.13 degrees. Accordingly, sunset will be at 11 Aries 13.

Finally, we can find the Ascendant in the Jamaspa system by simply adding the number of degrees that ascended over the horizon to the Sun's coordinates at sunrise:

53.85 + 191.13 = 244.98

Dividing the obtained number by 30 degrees will take us to the sign of Sagittarius, and the Ascendant will be in 4.98 degrees of Sagittarius. If the decimals are converted into minutes, we will obtain 4 Sagittarius 57.

(For your reference, the Ascendant in Western house systems for this data is 17 Scorpio 14.)

For those who enjoy formulas, here is one for a daytime birth:

$$\text{SUNsr} + \frac{(Tb - Tsr)}{(Tsr - Tss) / 180}$$

Where SUNsr is the coordinate of the Sun at sunrise:

Tb is the time of birth

Tsr is the time at sunrise

Tss is the time at sunset

In the next example we will consider the horoscope of a person born at night. We will again use Vancouver as the location with the data of June 5, 2007, at 1:05 a.m. In this case we need to determine the length of the night. On the given day the sunrise was at 5:10. We will also need the time of sunset on the previous day—that is, June 4. This will result in 21:12, with consideration being given to changes from Daylight Saving Time.

The length of the night = 24:00 − 21:12 + 5:10 = 7 hours, 58 minutes, or 478 minutes. The average speed of ascent of each degree V = 478 / 180 = 2.66 minutes.

To find how much time passed between sunset and the time of birth,

24:00 − 21:12 + 1:05 = 3 hours, 53 minutes, or 233 minutes.

How many degrees ascended over the horizon from the time of sunset until the time of birth?

233 / 2.66 = 87.59 degrees.

Now let's find the coordinates of the Sun at sunset (21:12 on June 4). The Sun must be in the Descendant in all Western house systems. We obtain 14.09', or in decimals, 14.15 of Gemini. Here we must note an exception: for those born at night we take the opposite degree: that is, 14.15 of Sagittarius, or 254.15 in a 360-degree format. Then we find the medical Ascendant.

254.15 + 87.59 = 341.74, or 11 Aquarius 44.

In a Western house system this will be the twenty-third degree of Aquarius.

The formula for a nighttime birth:

$$(\text{SUNss} - 180) + \frac{(Tb - Tss)}{(Tss - Tsr) / 180}$$

Where SUNss is the coordinate of the Sun at sunset:

Tb is the time of birth

Tss is the time at sunset

Tsr is the time at sunrise

After we find the medical Ascendant, the rest is easy because all houses are equal.

I understand that this process might appear tedious to modern astrologers—including myself—who are accustomed to the convenience of computers. As previously mentioned, some European astrological software programs have this medical house system and hopefully North American astrological programs will eventually adopt it.

The Houses of the Medical Chart

Each house of the medical chart has its own significance and characteristics. We will always pay attention to the sign in the house, as it will indicate a lack or excess of energy in the corresponding part of the body or organ. Also, the rule that the first house corresponds to Aries, the second to Taurus, the fifth to Leo, and so on must also be maintained. Accordingly, each house is tied to a specific part of the body or to an organ. Negative indicators in a house speak to a weakness of the corresponding organ or organs.

The *first house* is important because a person's initial reserve of strength is determined by it. Because it corresponds to the sign of Aries, it is responsible for indicators associated with the head.

The *second house* is associated with the biochemical processes of digestion. It is precisely by this house (with some other additions) that diet is determined. It is also associated with the throat and thyroid gland.

The *third house* is related to motor activity as well as the respiratory system. With an afflicted third house the lungs may be initially weak.

The *fourth house* is associated with the lymphatic system and is also an indicator of the presence of genetic diseases. An afflicted planet in the fourth house indicates genetic diseases, which are usually difficult to treat. One should also look at the sign on the cusp of the fourth house.

The *fifth house* is associated with the heart and the cardiovascular system in general. Here, illnesses caused by an idle life are also present.

The *sixth house* is one of the most important houses of the medical chart, and thus should be carefully examined. It indicates a person's susceptibility to illnesses. The sixth house determines simple illnesses with clear symptoms, which are easily treated with conventional medicine. Furthermore, the sign of the sixth house, especially its cusp, will indicate the form in which illnesses will progress. In this way Mars will point to an acute form of illness, while Saturn will signify a chronic form, and so on. The sixth house will also indicate industrial injuries and occupational diseases. This house, just as with the sign of Virgo, is associated with the intestines and will also be considered when determining a suitable diet.

The *seventh house* is related to the kidneys, the urinary system, and the endocrine system of the lower level (adrenal gland and prostate).

The *eighth house* indicates illnesses from external causes, as well as injuries, catastrophes, and their consequences. Here one can also find situations of extreme stress, critical situations with health, and surgical procedures. This house is associated with the reproductive organs. Women's infertility and men's sexual ability are determined by it.

The *ninth house* is related to the hips, hip joints, and liver function.

The *tenth house*, through analysis of the Midheaven, its sign and degree, can determine the aftereffects of illnesses. If at the time of the occurrence of an illness a difficult transit passed through the tenth house, the disease will likely be difficult to treat and might become chronic. The tenth house is also related to the spinal cord and the skeletal system. One must look out for afflicted planets in this house.

The *eleventh house* is related to the shins and is associated with the vascular system. New and unexpected illnesses can be found there.

The *twelfth house* is important and is related to illnesses with hidden symptoms. Generally, these illnesses are of a psychosomatic nature. They are more difficult to treat than the illnesses of the sixth house. Here, nontraditional medicine is more suitable. Negative planets in the twelfth house may bring mental illnesses. Because the twelfth house corresponds to the sign of Pisces, it is related to the feet but is not limited to them. It is associated with a person's whole body through the nervous system.

The Order of Houses Interpretation

Because medical houses don't have equal significance, the order below is the most effective in chart interpretation.

1. The first step is to look at the Ascendant and the first house as indicators of the basic vital force. Consider the sign, the degree of the Ascendant, and especially a planet on the Ascendant, if any. The orb for a conjunction with the Ascendant is ten degrees for the first house and five degrees for the twelfth. If the planet on the Ascendant is evil, then the illness associated with it could very well surface in the early years.

I do not agree with the opinion of some authors that the sign of the Ascendant is weakened and that there is a danger of illness associated with it. This only makes sense if the Ascendant is seriously afflicted by negative aspects. Illnesses of the Ascendant are always acquired (not inherited or karmic).

On the whole, if planets of the first house are not afflicted, their dignity is greatly increased. It is good to have many planets in the first house: they are indicators of the strongest organs. Good Jupiter in the first house shows a healthy liver for one's entire life, which magnificently cleanses the body. Apparently, those who drink alcohol excessively but do not suffer from liver cirrhosis, have Jupiter in the first house or as a Hyleg. The Moon in the first house brings a healthy stomach that can digest almost anything. All this is true only if there are no squares or oppositions to the planets in the first house.

Pay attention to the aspects between the Ascendant, the Sun, and the Moon. The positive aspects dramatically increase the chance that a person will be in good health and live long.

2. Next examine the sixth and the twelfth houses together. As already mentioned, the sixth house determines the simple illnesses, while the twelfth determines the more complex illnesses of a psychosomatic character or those arising from spiritual causes. Analyze the sign and the planets in the house. The planets are always more important than the sign. By looking at the sixth house we will find the form that the illness will develop for any given person. Conventional medicine successfully treats illnesses of the sixth house. For example, with a spinal cord illness and Saturn in the sixth house, one should definitely contact a physician, as he or she will be of help. However, given the same illness but with Saturn in the twelfth house, traditional medicine may not be able to provide suitable treatment.

The sixth house is also indicative of the illnesses we suffer because of our trivial attitude toward our health. If we paid more attention to preventive measures, we could avoid being ill. For example, I'm sitting hunched over the computer, typing this text. I fully understand that due to my evil Saturn in the sixth house and problems with my spine, I ought to get up and do some spinal exercises. However, I'm too lazy to do that, the result of which, no doubt, I will soon be made aware of.

One should pay attention to the psychological roots of illnesses caused by the twelfth house and tackle these first. Here, non-traditional medicine often helps.

Those that do not have planets in the sixth or twelfth houses can be considered lucky: they will not be subject to illnesses to the same extent as those who do.

3. Next take into account the fourth house as related to hereditary illnesses.

4. After that consider the eighth house, by which illnesses caused by injuries are determined. With a good eighth house, there might not be any injuries at all. However, I believe that aspects between Mars, Saturn, and Uranus are much more important in this case.

5. It also makes sense to look at the second house, which is responsible for nutrition. If it is afflicted, there may be illnesses caused by poisoning, intoxication, and metabolic imbalance. Choosing the right diet based on this house can correct the metabolism and as a result improve health.

6. If any other house has a planetary stellium, it should also be closely analyzed.

If there are no planets in the sixth and twelfth houses and the Sun and Moon have a positive aspect, then the person will be in good health. He or she will only attract quick-passing illnesses. It is especially remarkable when there is a gathering of planets that are not afflicted in the first and tenth houses. This confirms good health.

The Parses of the Medical Horoscope

Parses (or Arabian Parts, or Lots) are conditional points, calculated based on certain formulas. There are two main parses used in medical charts: the Pars of Health and the Pars of Disease. They show a person's ability to avoid illnesses or be susceptible to them.

The source of these two Arabian Parts is Pavel Globa's *Medical Astrology* (not available in English).

The Formula for the Pars of Disease (the ASC refers to the medical Ascendant) is:

For daytime birth: ASC + Moon - Saturn

For nighttime birth: ASC + Saturn - Moon

The Formula for the Pars of Health is:

For daytime birth: ASC + Sun - Jupiter

For nighttime birth: ASC + Jupiter - Sun

With the calculation of any parses, the formula changes depending on the time of birth, whether it's at night or during the day. An example of Pars calculation is shown in chapter seven.

The parses are considered from the point of view of the sign where they are located, the houses, and degrees. The Pars of Disease indicates the most vulnerable part of the body or organ. It is like a gate for all illnesses, a person's "Achilles heel." The organ to which this pars points can remain strong for a considerable time, but under the influence of even insignificant external factors it may fail. The illness may spread from this organ further into the body, affecting other organs and even entire vital systems.

The Pars of Health indicates the strongest organ. This is the spot from which treatment should begin. It is one of the strongest energy centers of the horoscope (although the Hyleg is more important) and when it is influenced, energy is given to the entire organism, aiding in the process of recovery. The Pars of Health is activated when it is involved in transit aspects. It begins to work dynamically when a transit planet goes through it and the organism's natural defenses are activated. It is good to know when these periods will occur in order to increase the effects of the transit through work with energy or acupuncture. These influences can supplant illnesses.

These two parses do not necessarily indicate an illness but are the bearers of the forces of destruction or creation within the organism.

Besides the two main parses, there are a number of additional ones. For example, each organ has its own pars, but I do not use organ parses in my practice because doing so can result in information overload. However, I will say a few of words about them, as they can help in specific cases when a treatment is being chosen for a specific illness.

The general formula for an organ pars is:

For daytime birth:

Organ Pars = ASC + the coordinates of the organ's planet - the coordinates of the ruler of the sixth house.

Medical Astrology for Healing

For nighttime birth:

> Organ Pars = ASC + the coordinates of the organ's planet - the coordinates of the ruler of the twelfth house.

Generally, the parses of the seven most important organs—consistent with the visible planets—are considered. Sun/heart, Jupiter/liver, Venus/kidneys, and so on (see chapter one). If the sixth and the twelfth houses are located in Scorpio, Aquarius, or Pisces, accordingly, we will take Pluto, Uranus, and Neptune as the rulers. For Virgo we will take Mercury (not Proserpina), and for Libra, use Venus.

The parses take on more significance when they are in conjunction with planets or fixed stars. The orb for conjunction with the pars is a half-degree (thirty minutes). It is also important to look at the characteristics of the degree that the pars is in, as well as its ruler. For instance, if the Pars of Liver is in the degree of the Moon, this suggests that the consequences of liver disease can negatively impact the gastrointestinal tract. If the Pars of Liver is located in the degree of Jupiter—the planet that rules the liver—the disease is localized only in the liver and will not spill over to the other organs.

With the presence of a specific illness it makes sense to pay attention to the transits that affect the pars of the affected organ.

Chapter Five

Degrees

Critical Positive and Negative Degrees

Characteristics of degrees in medical astrology differ from the description of the Sabian degrees. There are so-called critical degrees as well as diagnostic degrees. The reference for critical degrees is found in Pavel Globa's *Medical Astrology*.

Critical degrees can be positive or negative. Positive critical degrees are associated with creative energy: they improve the release of toxins and recovery from diseases. Negative degrees indicate intoxication and susceptibility to infections: i.e. are destructive indicators. A person with negative degrees in his or her horoscope becomes sick earlier than others during an epidemic. Destructive energies have a much stronger effect on his or her body. Negative critical degrees lower immunity; positive ones reinforce. Here we must also look at which organ the degree is responsible for. For example, if a critical degree is connected with the stomach, then the person may be subject to frequent illness from even harmless foods.

Critical degrees are taken into account if they consist of planets, parses, or houses cusps. Pars of Health in a negative critical degree may not work because the negative influence of the degree can block the positive energy of the pars. This is especially true if there are tense aspects to it. Likewise, the Pars of Disease located in a positive critical degree and suppressed by aspects loses its significance and shouldn't be considered in the diagnostics.

One more clarification: when we identify degrees, round up to the next whole number, such as the first degree for 0°45' or the thirtieth degree for 29°56'. The degrees shown are the original ones.

Positive critical degrees are:
- The fourth degree of Aries, Cancer, Libra, and Capricorn
- The nineteenth degree of Taurus, Leo, Scorpio, and Aquarius
- The twenty-eighth degree of Gemini, Virgo, Sagittarius, and Pisces

Negative critical degrees are:
- The first degree of Aries, Cancer, Libra, and Capricorn
- The twelfth degree of Taurus, Leo, Scorpio, and Aquarius
- The twenty-fifth degree of Gemini, Virgo, Sagittarius, and Pisces

The connection to the negative degree weakens the planet. A positive critical degree, on the contrary, strengthens the characteristics of a planet it conjoins. If a critical degree is located on the cusp of the house, it is connected to the whole house: positive for positive degrees, and negative for negative degrees.

The presence of critical degrees on the cusps of the sixth and twelfth houses is especially important, remarkably so if their cusps are in positive degrees. If the sixth house has no planets and it starts with a critical positive degree, such a person would not be afflicted by disease and disease will not play any role in his or her life. If the twelfth house has positive degrees (in the absence of affliction), then the person is not mentally associated with disease and can independently remove the spiritual cause of disease. If the positive degree is on the cusp of the fourth house, even in the presence of unpleasant indicators in this house, the person can cope with genetic diseases because he or she will have a large influx of energy from the outside.

Critical degrees mostly determine external factors influencing health.

Diagnostic Degrees

Degrees by themselves are *never* an indicator of a disease. Other factors need to be taken into consideration, such as aspects, affliction, and planet status. Degrees only indicate the possibility of a disease and provide additional information, but negative aspects and evil planets predispose to illness. Thus, the main diagnostic degrees are:

Aries
1°: brain
3°: kidneys
5°: eyes
6°: meningitis
7°: endocrine system illnesses
8°: hair loss that accompanies the main disease
10°: blood disorders
11°: heart attack
13°: nervous disorders
14°: decay of tooth enamel
15°: parietal part of the brain

17°: overstrain and insomnia
20°: liver illnesses
21°: hearing loss; auditory nerves; tinnitus
23°: toothache; inflammation of the periosteum
24°: eyes
25°: eyes
28°: possibility of a heart attack
29°: subcortical layer of the brain
30°: delirium; fevers

Taurus
1°: esophagus
3°: larynx
4°: lungs
6°: endocrine system
7°: trachea
8°: neck (osteochondrosis; cervical myositis)
10°: vocal chords
12°: throat
13°: tonsils
14°: kidneys
15°: upper part of the stomach
17°: blood
18°: lungs
20°: parathyroid gland
21°: thyroid
24°: osteochondrosis
25°: lungs
27°: bronchi
29°: lungs

Gemini
3°: respiratory system
5°: hands

6°: forearms
7°: shoulders
13°: autonomic nervous system
15°: liver
16°: autonomic nervous system
18°: left lung
19°: right lung
20°: neuroses
23°: blood disorders
24°: sleep disturbances
26°: sexual perversion
29°: neurological disorders
30°: blood disorders

Cancer
2°: internal swelling
3°: hearing
4°: endocrine illnesses
8°: ears
9°: lungs
11°: eardrum; middle ear
13°: stomach; psychosomatics
14°: stomach
15°: stomach
17°: delirium; neuroses
18°: liver
22°: gallbladder; psychosomatics
23°: chronic appendicitis
24°: intestines
28°: schizophrenia

Leo
1°: heart
2°: aorta; major arteries
3°: medulla oblongata
5°: lens; eyeball

8°: heart; blood
9°: heart attack
13°: heart; thoracic spine
14°: spinal cord (meningitis)
15°: spinal cord
18°: spine
19°: hypertension
20°: hypertension
23°: skin (psoriasis)
30°: premature aging; impotence; frigidity

Virgo
6°: hernia
10°: liver
11°: gastrointestinal disorders
14°: blood disorders
15°: heart attack
18°: peritoneum; peritonitis
19°: sepsis
21°: appendicitis
22°: duodenum
23°: gastrointestinal disorders
27°: gastrointestinal disorders

Libra
4°: homeostasis of the organism as a whole
5°: endocrine illnesses
6°: kidneys
8°: heart
13°: bladder
14°: left adrenal gland
15°: right adrenal gland
16°: left kidney
17°: right kidney
22°: thyroid
23, 24, and 25°: possibility of sexual perversions

29°: spine
30°: small of the back (sciatica)

Scorpio
1°: urethra
2°: kidneys; bladder
3°: hemorrhoids; possibility of sexual perversion
5°: ovaries
7°: neurological disorders
8°: sexual perversions
11°: neurological disorders
15°: hair loss
17°: rectum
18°: endocrine illnesses
21°: genitals
22°: neurological disorders
27°: hair loss
29°: uterus; prostate gland

Sagittarius
1°: blood
2°: liver
11°: liver
12°: increased sexuality
13°: lungs
14°: spine
17°: liver
19°: heart
20°: liver
21°: blood
24°: blood; heart
26°: liver
30°: liver

Capricorn
2°: tooth decay; thrombosis
5°: metabolic disorder; salt deposit

7°: heart
8°: blood
9°: gastrointestinal disorders
11°: hematopoietic system
13°: gastrointestinal disorders
15°: teeth; gums
16°: joints
19°: teeth
20°: teeth
23°: hernias
25°: spleen
27°: lungs
28°: spine

Aquarius

2°: myopia; strabismus; retina; iris
4°: neurological disorders
5°: heart
6°: blood
7°: lungs
9°: lungs
10°: endocrine system
11°: mental illnesses
14°: medulla oblongata
16°: paralysis
17°: arthritis
18°: lungs
28°: shins

Pisces

3°: neurological disorders
6°: blood
9°: lungs
10°: feet (flat-footedness)
11°: blood
13°: tendency to alcoholism

14°: gastrointestinal disorders
16°: kidneys
19°: eczema and skin allergy
20°: medical intoxication
21°: hair loss that accompanies the main disease
23°: neurological disorders
26°: blood
27°: endocrine illnesses
29°: drug addiction

As is evident, degrees are directly related to the classification of organs according to the zodiac signs. Degrees of the liver are thus mainly located in Sagittarius, degrees of sexual organs in Scorpio, degrees of the stomach in Cancer, etc.

Once again, remember that degrees do not bring disease; they provide additional information to the clinical picture.

Passive Degrees

There is also a concept of passive degrees, which comes from Indian astrology. The information revealed by passive degrees is different from that of diagnostic, active degrees. Active degrees are those that have planets and house cusps. Passive degrees are those with which the planets form the main aspects: square, opposition, sextile and trine.

We pay attention to the passive degrees only if there is a specific disease because these degrees do not indicate a disease but rather its implications or possible complications after the disease. For example, if the Sun is located in the third degree of Aquarius, the passive degree for the square will be the third of Taurus. If transiting Mars will pass through the third of Taurus, it can cause a bad cold or infection (with additional indicators). In this case the third degree of Taurus is a degree of Jupiter, which suggests that antibiotics should not be overused during the illness because the liver could suffer.

Knowing the characteristics of a passive degree, we can consider preventive measures to avoid complications. If it is the liver, think about diet; if it is eyes, do not overwork the vision during an illness; if it is the heart, use supporting medicine, etc. It makes sense to pre-calculate the passive degrees. There are only seven for each planet: two squares, two sextiles, two trines, and one opposition.

Chapter Six

Fixed Stars

Fixed stars play a fairly big role in a medical chart. They don't indicate diseases by themselves but add inevitability if illnesses are confirmed by other factors. The importance of stars greatly increases if they are in conjunction with luminaries or an Ascendant. Conjunctions with other planets, angular points, and two main parses also need to be taken into consideration.

As usual, we take a projection of fixed stars on the ecliptic, and in calculating their coordinates we always add precession. Precession is the movement of the axis of the equator with the speed of one degree in seventy-two years. The necessary amendments can be found with the help of simple calculations.

Medical astrology considers stars of the 1st, 2nd and 3rd magnitude. Orbs for a conjunction with a star are: 1st magnitude, thirty minutes; 2nd magnitude, twenty minutes; and 3rd magnitude, ten minutes.

We also take nebulas into consideration. Stars may have both a negative and positive influence (depending on the star), but the influence of nebulas is always negative in medical astrology. Nebulas are especially malicious for senses—vision in particular—if the Sun and the Moon are in conjunction with them. The orb for nebulas is twenty minutes.

Fixed stars in a medical chart are more important than degrees. If a positive star falls into a bad degree, it obliterates the degree's destructive characteristic and vice versa: a negative star can negate any positive degree. Following are the coordinates of main stars and nebulas significant in medical astrology, together with their magnitude and a short description of their influence. The descriptions are according to Pavel Globa's *Medical Astrology*. Star coordinates are from the year 2000.

Negative Fixed Stars

1. Algenib. 2nd magnitude. 9 Aries 09. Gives bleeding, wounds, and sepses.
2. Sharatan. 2nd magnitude. 5 Taurus 58. Skin diseases.

3. Hamal. 2nd magnitude. 7 Taurus 39. Headaches, migraine. On the level of spiritual diseases, cruelty and aggressiveness.

4. Algol. 1st magnitude. 26 Taurus10. On the medical level it shows a possibility of poisoning and a tendency toward drug addiction and alcoholism. This is the most malicious of all fixed stars.

5. Aldebaran. 1st magnitude. 9 Gemini 47. Stroke, kidney disease, and clotting of blood.

6. Rigel. 1st magnitude. 16 Gemini 49. Negatively influences limbs, joints, and the motor system.

7. Bellatrix. 1st magnitude. 20 Gemini 56. In conjunction with the Sun or Moon it contributes to blindness. In conjunction with other planets it may affect the spinal cord. If this star is conjunct Pluto it could be associated with brain tumors.

8. Capella. 1st magnitude. 21 Gemini 51. Schizophrenia, kleptomania.

9. Polaris (Kinosura). 2nd magnitude. 28 Gemini 34. Gives general weakness and low immunity.

10. Betelgeuze. 1st magnitude. 28 Gemini 48. Salt deposit in joints, fractures and injuries.

11. Tejat. 3rd magnitude. 3 Cancer 26. Affects the sexual system and often gives manias.

12. Alhena. 2nd magnitude. 9 Cancer 06. Negative influence to legs.

13. Sirius. 0 magnitude. The brightest star in the sky. It has the biggest orb: 40 minutes. 14 Cancer 04. Poisoning.

14. Wasat. 3rd magnitude. 18 Cancer 31. Illness from poisons, toxins, and gases.

15. Castor. 1st magnitude. 20 Cancer 14. Difficulty in the healing of wounds and increased risk of thromboses, inner bleeding, and injuries to legs and arms.

16. North Donkey, 7 Leo 32, and South Donkey, 8 Leo 43. Both have 3rd magnitude. They have a negative influence on the male reproductive cells and very occasionally on the female cells.

17. Alphard. 2nd magnitude. 27 Leo 16. It has a negative influence on the cardio-vascular system and indicates arrhythmia, heart attack, and stroke.

18. Zosma. 2nd magnitude. 11 Virgo 18. Poisoning and disorders of the alimentary tract.

19. Denibola. 2nd magnitude. 21 Virgo 37. Indicates destruction of the immune and endocrine systems.

20. Vindemiatrix. 2nd magnitude. 9 Libra 56. Negative influence on backbone, legs, and the sexual sphere.

21. Caphir. 3rd magnitude. 10 Libra 20. Festering wounds and leprosy.

22. Algorab. 2nd magnitude. 13 Libra 26. Gangrene, festering wounds, leprosy and tendency to formation of tumors.

23. Arcturus. 1st magnitude. 24 Libra 13. This is the star of venereal diseases and sexual perversity. Illnesses of adrenal glands are also possible.

24. Khambalia. 3rd magnitude. 10 Scorpio 07. Has a negative influence on the blood formula.

25. Zubenelgenubi (Kiffa Australis). 2nd magnitude. 15 Scorpio 04. General weakening in health and vitality.

26. Unukalhai. 2nd magnitude. 22 Scorpio 04. Affects the immune system.

27. Antares. 1st magnitude. 9 Sagittarius 25. Inclination to manias, phobias, and self-destruction. Poisonings.
28. Rasalhague. 2nd magnitude. 21 Sagittarius 23. Liver diseases: hepatitis and cirrhosis.
29. Lesath. 2nd magnitude. 24 Sagittarius 00. Negative influence on mentality.
30. Terebellum. 4th magnitude (four-minute orb). 25 Sagittarius 51. The liver.
31. Bos. 3rd magnitude. 5 Aquarius 09. The nervous system.
32. Armus. 3rd magnitude. 12 Aquarius 35. Rupture, piles, and problems with the pelvis.
33. Castra. 3rd magnitude. 20 Aquarius 11. The sexual sphere.
34. Sadalsuud. 2nd magnitude. 23 Aquarius 23. Negative influence for the heart.
35. Skat. 3rd magnitude. 8 Pisces 52. Mentality. The star of epilepsy.
36. Markab. 2nd magnitude. 23 Pisces 29. Fevers and wounds difficult to cure.
37. Scheat. 2nd magnitude. 29 Pisces 22. Negative for blood and liver. Also can indicate hysteria and personality disorders.

Please note that information about fixed stars on the medical level and the level of events can be very different. For example, Arcturus is a great star on the level of events but the same cannot be said about its influence in human health.

Positive Fixed Stars

1. Regulus. 1st magnitude. 29 Leo 49. Indicates a stronger heart.
2. Labrum. 2nd magnitude. 26 Virgo 41. In general, this is a powerful star of healing. It is wonderful for energy healers.
3. Spica. 1st magnitude. 23 Libra 50. Strengthened immune system.
4. Vega. 1st magnitude. 15 Capricorn 18. Improved thought processes and strengthened the liver and haematogenic functions.
5. Altair. 1st magnitude. 1 Aquarius 46. Stronger lungs and nervous system. Also an asset in curing infectious diseases.
6. Fomalhaut. 1st magnitude. 3 Pisces 51. Stronger mind and higher energy. Prolonged youth and increased male potency.

Nebulas

1. Andromeda Nebula (or Galaxi). 27 Aries 50. Has a strong influence on eyesight and other senses. With the presence of this nebula, diseases of the eyes always have an unpredictable course and have unclear and changing symptoms. If Mercury is in conjunction with the nebula it indicates allergies.
2. Pleiades (Seven Sisters). Its main star, Alcyone, has a projection of 29 Taurus 59. In general this nebula goes from 29 Taurus 24 to 0 Gemini 05. It indicates impairment of all senses, but eyesight suffers the most. In conjunction with the Sun or Moon it may indicate glaucoma or even blindness. In conjunction with Saturn it indicates deafness; with Mercury it might influence the lungs.

3. Hyades. 5 Gemini 42. Senses.

4. Ensis. Nebula in the Orion constellation. 22 Gemini 59. Senses.

5. Milky Way. We pay attention to only two points where the Milky Way crosses the ecliptic: south crossing, 27 Gemini 35; north crossing, 29 Sagittarius 39. Bad influence for eyesight, hearing, and nervous system. May indicate a weakening of memory along with accelerated aging and low vitality. Sometimes can indicate to paralysis. It has an especially malicious influence if it is on Ascendant.

6. Beehive Cluster (or Praesepe). 7 Leo 23. Problems with eyesight. Also can indicate mental diseases and drug addiction.

7. Copula. 25 Virgo 07. Indicates poor eyesight and hearing; may affect optic nerve. Can indicate auditory hallucinations and deafness.

8. Aculeus. 25 Sagittarius 46. Impaired senses, especially the sense of smell. Can indicate strong and incurable allergies as well as epilepsy.

9. Facies. 8 Capricorn 18. Negative influence on senses.

Via Combusta

There is an area in the zodiac that can weaken all planets despite their strength and status in a horoscope: the Via Combusta. Located between the eighteenth and thirtieth degrees of Libra, in mythology this is the area of Phaeton's destruction, and the hypothetical planet Juno exploded in this area (not to be confused with the asteroid). The Sun comes transits this area from October 11 to 23 every year, when many people might experience lower vitality. Even Hyleg and Antihyleg lose a bit of their power when they fall into these degrees.

Via Combusta doesn't change with precession. It is related to the disappearance of the mass of accumulated negative energy in the solar system. The place where Juno should have been is considered unfavorable.

These are the general concepts about Via Combusta but I've been unable to find any confirmation of its negative role in my practice. I use Via Combusta only in horary astrology, not in medical astrology. You can investigate this for yourself to see if it works.

Chapter Seven

The Hyleg and the Antihyleg

Determining the Two Main Planets of the Medical Chart

The concept of the Hyleg was introduced by Arab astrologers. Hyleg indicates the strongest organ, through which the main flow of energy travels to the body. The Hyleg can determine the initial reserve of a person's vitality, how long it will last and whether the person will be resistant to illness. It may be that the Hyleg and Antihyleg are the most important indicators in the medical horoscope.

In principle, any planet can be in the role of the Hyleg. However, first we must draw attention to the Sun and Moon. Ancient Arab astrologers believed that in the male horoscope the Hyleg was the Sun, and in the female the Moon. Hindu astrologer Jamaspa introduced an amendment to this. He believed that in order to occupy the position of the Hyleg, the Sun and/or the Moon must not be located in negative critical degrees and must occupy special Hyleg places.

Hyleg places are the angular points of the chart: Ascendant, Descendant, Midheaven, and IC. The orb for angular houses is ten degrees; and for cadent houses, it is five degrees. If the Sun and the Moon are located in Hyleg places, additional circumstances need to be considered. The male horoscope with a daytime birth has its Hyleg in the Sun. For the female horoscope with a daytime birth, the Hyleg is the Moon. For nighttime births the opposite is true: the Hyleg for males is the Moon, and for females it is the Sun. Of course this is an accurate description only if they are located on the angular points and not in the negative critical degrees. The Hyleg can be in critical positive degrees.

The concept of the Antihyleg was used only by Hindu astrologers. Generally, the Antihyleg is opposite of the Hyleg. The planet Antihyleg is a destroyer of good health; it shows the organ that may be the first to become susceptible, the one that all the other illnesses will pass through. The aspects of the Antihyleg with other planets will indicate the organs and systems to which the negative energy can transfer.

The Antihyleg can also be any planet. The planets that indicate "big" and "little" disasters—Saturn and Mars—are the first to be considered. The rule for these is the same: they can be the Antihyleg only if they are located at angular points. The orbs are the same as mentioned above. It is believed that for men born in daytime the Antihyleg is Mars and that for women with a daytime birth it is Saturn. For nighttime births it is the opposite: Saturn for men and Mars for women.

The Hyleg and the Antihyleg are always considered together in order to identify which is stronger and how it impacts the general health of a person. If the Hyleg is stronger than the Antihyleg, then a person will possess significant powers of recovery that will aid in quickly managing any illness. If the Hyleg and Antihyleg are connected by an aspect, this may radically change the clinical picture of the illness. For example, if the Hyleg Sun is in a trine aspect with the Antihyleg Mars (and Hyleg is stronger), it can be said that the powers of the Sun will reduce the acuteness of any illness caused by Mars. For healers using non-traditional medicine, the knowledge of these two main planets can prove extremely valuable, enabling the choice of the most effective treatment method.

If the Hyleg and Antihyleg are not identifiable by the simple rules described above (use of the Sun, Moon, Mars, and/or Saturn), they can be found through the Tables of Dignities.

Tables of Dignities

The Tables of Dignities are used not only for finding the Hyleg and Antihyleg but also for determining the points—positive or negative—that the other planets have. The medical status of planets is necessary for the diagnosis of complex illnesses. As discussed previously, the simpler illnesses can be seen using only the aspects and location of planets in signs and houses. But what if a person has an illness related to a specific planet but that planet is not afflicted by anything and has only positive aspects? In this case, it is certain that the planet has a negative status.

Conditionally, the planets are divided into good and evil. The good, creative planets are a source of energy, while the evil, destructive planets indicate weak spots in the organism. There are also neutral planets. In order to determine whether the planet has good or evil power, the Tables of Dignities are consulted. There are two of them: one for the Hyleg and one for the Antihyleg. They are, however, considered together.

The Tables of Dignities include seven columns. The indicators that play the main part in determining the Hyleg and the Antihyleg, regardless of whether they are planets, parses or the cusps of houses, are recorded in the first column.

For the Hyleg we consider the Sun, Moon, cusp of the sixth house, planet closest to the Midheaven (MC) from the eastern side, and the Pars of Health.

For the Antihyleg we consider Mars, Saturn, cusp of the twelfth house, planet closest to the IC from the western side, and the Pars of Disease. Readers are reminded that the cusps of all the houses are in the medical system of Jamaspa.

Tables of Dignities						
Planets	Coordinate	Sign Ruler	Exaltation	Degree Ruler	Term Ruler	Decan Ruler
Hyleg	Points (+)	5	4	3	2	1
Sun						
Moon						
Sixth Cusp						
Planet around MC						
Pars of Health						
Antihyleg	Points (−)	5	4	3	2	1
Mars						
Saturn						
Twelfth Cusp						
Planet around IC						
Pars of Disease						

In the second column the coordinates of the points from the first column are entered.

The third column has the rulers of the signs where the planets, parses, and cusps are located, that is:

Aries-Mars	Leo-Sun	Sagittarius-Jupiter
Taurus-Venus	Virgo-Proserpina and Mercury	Capricorn-Saturn
Gemini-Mercury	Libra-Chiron and Venus	Aquarius-Uranus and Saturn
Cancer-Moon	Scorpio-Pluto and Mars	Pisces-Neptune and Jupiter

The fourth column contains the planets that exalt in the indicated signs.

Aries-Sun	Leo-Pluto	Sagittarius-Jupiter
Taurus-Moon	Virgo-Mercury	Capricorn-Mars
Gemini-Proserpina	Libra-Saturn	Aquarius-Neptune
Cancer-Jupiter	Scorpio-Uranus	Pisces-Venus

The last three columns are for the degree rulers, terms rulers and decan rulers. The division of the zodiac into the terms (five degrees) and decans (ten degrees) is used by ancient Hindu and European astrologers. However, their rulers, just like the degree rulers, are different from those used in general astrology.

Degree rulers are divided in the following way:

Medical Astrology for Healing

For Aries, Gemini, Leo, Libra, Sagittarius and Aquarius, the first degree of the sign is ruled by Mars, the second by Venus, the third by Mercury, the fourth by the Moon, the fifth by the Sun, the sixth by Proserpina, the seventh by Chiron, the eighth by Pluto, the ninth by Jupiter, the tenth by Saturn, the eleventh by Uranus, the twelfth by Neptune, the thirteenth again by Mars, the fourteenth again by Venus, and so on. The thirtieth degree is ruled by Proserpina.

For Taurus, Cancer, Virgo, Scorpio, Capricorn and Pisces, the ruler of the first degree is Chiron, the second is ruled by Pluto, the third by Jupiter, the fourth by Saturn, the fifth by Uranus, the sixth by Neptune, the seventh by Mars, the eighth by Venus, the ninth by Mercury, the tenth by the Moon, the eleventh by the Sun, and the twelfth by Proserpina, the thirteenth again by Chiron, and so on. The last degree is ruled by Neptune.

The countdown of terms and decans begins from 0 Aries. The zodiac counts seventy-two terms, each of five degrees. The terms rulers are in this order: the first by Mars, the second by Venus, the third by Mercury, the fourth by the Moon, the fifth by the Sun, the sixth by Proserpina, the seventh by Chiron, the eighth by Pluto, the ninth by Jupiter, the tenth by Saturn, the eleventh by Uranus, the twelfth by Neptune, the thirteenth again by Mars, and so on. The last term (from 26 to 30 Pisces) is ruled by Neptune.

It is easier to calculate the decan rulers. They are constructed on the principle of the trine of elements; for instance, the trine of fire. For the first decan, the ruler of the first sign of the element is selected; for the second decan, the ruler of the second sign of the same element is selected; and so on. For example, for the trine of fire (Aries, Leo, and Sagittarius), the decan rulers for Aries are: 1 to 10 degrees, Mars; 11 to 20 degrees, the Sun (which rules Leo), 21 to 30 degrees, Jupiter (which rules Sagittarius). If the sign has two rulers, we take only the higher planet, including Proserpina for Virgo and Chiron for Libra.

The table on the next page can be used for your convenience.

The rulers of all the terms, decans, and degrees can be found in Appendix 2.

After filling out the table we can add a little bit of math, namely the calculation of the points of each planet. We can see from the table how many points each column received from five to one (descending). The sum from the table of the Hyleg is considered with a plus sign, and from the table of the Antihyleg with a minus sign. We compare the two resulting sums and subtract the least from the greatest. As a result, we obtain a general point for each planet, which can be positive, negative or zero. Planets with a positive point are considered good, while planets with a negative point are evil; planets with a point of zero are neutral. It is also important to look at how great the total result is. If it is plus or minus one, the planet can also be considered neutral. Neutral planets do not carry any charge; however, they cannot be considered positive, as with difficult transiting aspects directed to them, they can act as triggers.

The planet with the maximum number of positive points will be the Hyleg, and the one with the most negative ones the Antihyleg. This is the case if the Sun, Moon, Mars, or Saturn is not located

Decan Rulers			
Zodiac Sign	*1st Decan*	*2nd Decan*	*3rd Decan*
Aries	Mars	Sun	Jupiter
Taurus	Venus	Proserpina	Saturn
Gemini	Mercury	Chiron	Uranus
Cancer	Moon	Pluto	Neptune
Leo	Sun	Jupiter	Mars
Virgo	Proserpina	Saturn	Venus
Libra	Chiron	Uranus	Mercury
Scorpio	Pluto	Neptune	Moon
Sagittarius	Jupiter	Mars	Sun
Capricorn	Saturn	Venus	Proserpina
Aquarius	Uranus	Mercury	Chiron
Pisces	Neptune	Moon	Pluto

near an angular points of the horoscope.

There is an additional consideration relating to the lunar nodes. The conjunction with the North Node (Rahu) increases the planet's strength by five points, regardless of whether it is good or evil. The conjunction of the South Node (Ketu) with a planet decreases its good or evil power by five points. The orb for conjunction is six degrees for the seven visible planets and five degrees for the others.

If the Hyleg and the Antihyleg are found before the tables are constructed, a certain number of points also has to be added. If the Sun and the Moon are in Hyleg points, add twelve points to those planets if they are in eastern houses (one, two, three, ten, eleven, or twelve) and ten points if they are in western (four, five, six, seven, eight, or nine). We add these to the table of Hyleg with a plus sign. The same goes for Saturn and Mars if they are located at angular points: twelve points if they are eastern and ten if they are western. Add these to the table of Antihyleg with a minus sign.

It is very important to compare the power of the Hyleg and the Antihyleg, as this will show the individual's level of health and resistance to illness. It may also be of benefit to compare the sum of the points of the negative and positive planets.

The subject of this chapter is quite complex, and an example is included at the end of this chapter to clarify the procedure.

Planets in the Role of the Hyleg

Sun

A person with a Hyleg Sun has a large reserve of vitality. The Sun brings vital energy to the rest of the organs. This person will have an excellent resistance to illnesses. If the Hyleg is stronger than the Antihyleg, then the person will not experience illness early in life. As well, a Hyleg Sun indicates a completely healthy cardiovascular system. However, if the Hyleg is weaker than the Antihyleg, the Sun energies will not last and the person could suffer from a variety of illnesses. The organism can slowly degenerate but the heart will remain healthy to the end.

Moon

A strong Moon brings a healthy gastro-intestinal system, non-problematic blood circulation, and a well-functioning endocrine system. A person with a Moon Hyleg has an incredible sensitivity toward his or her health. The individual can sense the onset of illness and even block it using psychological energy. People like this are excellent at healing themselves through self-hypnosis. And again, if the Moon is weaker than the Antihyleg, then anything other than the intestine can become ill.

Mercury

In the role of the Hyleg, Mercury strengthens the lungs and autonomic nervous system. This person is insured against bronchitis, pneumonia, and asthma. Furthermore, Mercury brings heightened motor activity.

Venus

A strong Venus brings well-functioning kidneys and the entire urinary tract. The main energy center will be in the kidneys. Nothing threatens the thyroid gland, as well as the rest of the endocrine system (provided that the Moon and Neptune, that are also responsible for the work of the endocrine system, are favorable). If the Antihyleg is stronger, then it may happen that there will only be enough energy for the support of the kidney function.

Mars

A strong Mars brings a well-developed muscular system. A person with Hyleg Mars will not experience muscle sprains, overstrain, insomnias, headaches, or fevers. Mars is responsible for the head, which will be healthy.

Jupiter

Hyleg Jupiter brings a strong, healthy liver. The liver is considered to be a person's "animal" soul. The main energy center will be located there. The person will have excellent vitality, which will flow not from the heart but from the liver. If the Antihyleg is stronger than Jupiter, then the liver itself will be healthy, but the organs related to it may suffer: the stomach and the gallbladder. This may also affect the blood.

Saturn

I have never encountered a Saturn Hyleg; however, it is theoretically possible. The information related to the Hyleg can be useful to describe planets with a positive status. Saturn Hyleg brings a well-functioning skeletal system, strong teeth, well-adjusted gallbladder, and an absence of fractures. The energy center in this case will be the spleen, which is why it is contraindicated for a person with Saturn Hyleg to have the spleen removed, as it serves as the source of his or her

life energy.

Uranus

The energy center here is the cerebellum, which is responsible for coordination. A person with Uranus Hyleg will not suffer from illnesses of the autonomic nervous system; his or her tendons, ligaments and joints will be in order. However, if Uranus is weaker than the Antihyleg, problems with the nervous system are a possibility and could include neuroses and hysteric episodes.

Neptune

This person will have a well-functioning pancreas. It is the energy center and supports the function of the entire endocrine system. The person's psyche will also be normal (but it is necessary to consider other indicators).

Pluto

A strong Pluto that does not have any negative aspects brings the absence of cancer, as well as chances of internal bleeding. For men the energy center is the prostate and for women it is the uterus.

Proserpina

Because Proserpina is connected to the immune system, those who have it as the Hyleg will have excellent immunity and will not suffer from epidemics. The energy center is the eyes. It is believed that Proserpina is responsible for the left eye and the not-yet-discovered Vulcan for the right eye (in the meantime, the Moon is responsible for the right eye.)

Chiron

I have never encountered Chiron as the Hyleg and its role in this regard is not well understood.

The Hyleg does not bring full deliverance from an illness. It is necessary to consider all its aspects. If, for example, the Hyleg is in the centre of a T-square, then the illnesses of the organ ruled by the Hyleg can occur from time to time but will be short term and without aftereffects.

The Planets in the Role of the Antihyleg

Sun

The Sun as the Antihyleg brings a lack of vitality as well as an initial physical weakness. The cardiovascular system suffers. There is a possibility of heart attack.

Moon

The stomach and the entire gastro-intestinal system are weakened. This person is very sensitive to all toxins and foods of poor quality. This manifests particularly in the younger years. However, if the Hyleg is stronger than the Antihyleg, with age all the symptoms may permanently disappear.

Mercury

The lungs and respiratory system in general are weakened. It is important to watch closely the condition of the respiratory system for children with a Mercury Antihyleg.

Venus

This indicates an initial weakness of the kidneys and bladder. The endocrine system suffers, especially the thyroid gland.

Mars

The main weak spot is the head. All illnesses infiltrate through the head. Illnesses may be very serious, such as meningitis with an affliction of the entire nervous system. Less severe cases are also possible, such as sprains of muscles and ligaments, or unpleasant, but not deadly, hemorrhoids. There is also a great possibility of anemia, as Mars is responsible for the level of hemoglobin.

Jupiter

In this case not only the liver but also the "animal" soul of the person suffers. This person does not lose vitality, which is ruled by the Sun, but rather the possession of life forces, thereby becoming listless and inert.

Saturn

Saturn Antihyleg causes serious problems with the bones, including joints. Teeth can be ruined. Negative aspects with Mars could bring about frequent fractures. There is a great probability of gallstones and kidney stones. The function of the spinal cord may be disrupted, which can lead to blood diseases, even leukemia.

Uranus

Uranus Antihyleg disrupts the coordination of movement, brings about problems with blood pressure, neurosis, nervous ticks, and a state of convulsion. If there is a negative aspect with Saturn, Parkinson's disease may arise. The chance of stroke increases.

Neptune

The psyche suffers greatly. The endocrine system is also weakened, especially the pancreas. If there are negative aspects with Venus and the Moon, diabetes may develop.

Pluto

Predisposes to tumors.

Proserpina

Proserpina Antihyleg brings about a sudden decrease in immunity. The person is prone to all infectious diseases, including the exotic kind. There is a likelihood of skin diseases and sexually transmitted infections. Eyebrows and eyelashes may start to fall out.

Chiron

Chiron has not been studied as an Antihyleg.

As mentioned previously, the Antihyleg is the source of destruction. However, if the Hyleg is stronger than the Antihyleg, then the weak organ can be strengthened and cured. Generally, the illnesses of the Antihyleg manifest themselves in the early years. Nevertheless, these illnesses may disappear later on (if the power of the Hyleg is used properly).

Complex illnesses can be revealed with the help of the Tables of Dignities. Symptoms do not always paint an accurate picture of an illness; sometimes a less severe illness emerges and frees a person from a more serious illness. For example, with Saturn Antihyleg, skin afflictions may develop, but these may spare the person from a bone marrow illness, which is often fatal. It's important to be very careful with symptoms. If one attempts to cure them, then the illness may pass, but it may trigger more serious illnesses.

Medical astrology allows a holistic approach that can find hidden causes of illness and offer insight into curing the organism, not the symptoms.

A Sample Construction of the Tables of Dignities

Looking at Figure 2 on the next page, the medical Ascendant is located at 19 Scorpio. Because the system of houses is equilateral, all the houses begin in the nineteenth degree. Some of these are positive critical degrees.

Next we will find the Pars of Health and the Pars of Disease. The person was born during daytime so we use the daytime birth formula (see Chapter 4).

Pars of Health = 228°41' + 71°13' - 45°50' = 254°04' or the 15th degree of Sagittarius

Pars of Disease = 228°41' + 112°33' - 119°38' = 221°36' or the 12th degree of Scorpio

Now we can begin the construction of the Tables of Dignities.

Planets	Coordinate	Sign Ruler	Exaltation	Degree Ruler	Term Ruler	Decan Ruler
Hyleg	*Points (+)*	*5*	*4*	*3*	*2*	*1*
Sun	12 Gem	Mer	Pro	Nep	Mer	Chi
The Moon	23 Can	Mo	Jup	Su	Ura	Nep
Sixth Cusp	19 Ari	Mar	Su	Chi	Mo	Su
Planet around MC	10 Lib	Ven, Chi	Sat	Sat	Ven	Chi
Pars of Health	15 Sag	Jup	Chi	Mer	Mer	Mar
Antihyleg	*Points (-)*	*5*	*4*	*3*	*2*	*1*
Mars	10 Leo	Su	Plu	Sat	Ven	Su
Saturn	30 Can	Mo	Jup	Nep	Nep	Nep
Twelfth Cusp	19 Lib	Ven, Chi	Sat	Chi	Mo	Ura
Planet around IC	1 Tau	Ven	Mo	Chi	Chi	Ven
Pars of Disease	12 Sco	Plu	Ura	Pro	Jup	Nep

The planet closest to the Midheaven from the eastern side is Pluto, and the planet closest to the IC from the western side is Chiron.

After filling in all the columns we calculate the points.

Su	Mo	Mer	Ven	Mar	Jup	Sat	Ura	Nep	Plu	Pro	Chi
+8	+7	+12	+7	+6	+9	+7	+2	+4	0	+4	+14
-6	-11	0	-13	0	-6 -5	-7	-5	-7	-9	-3	-13
+2	-4	+12a	-6	+6a	-2	0	-3	-3	-9a	+1	+1

"-5" is added to Jupiter because it is connected to the South Node. Mars is very close to the angular point (Midheaven) but not close enough to be considered the Antihyleg because it is in a cadent house.

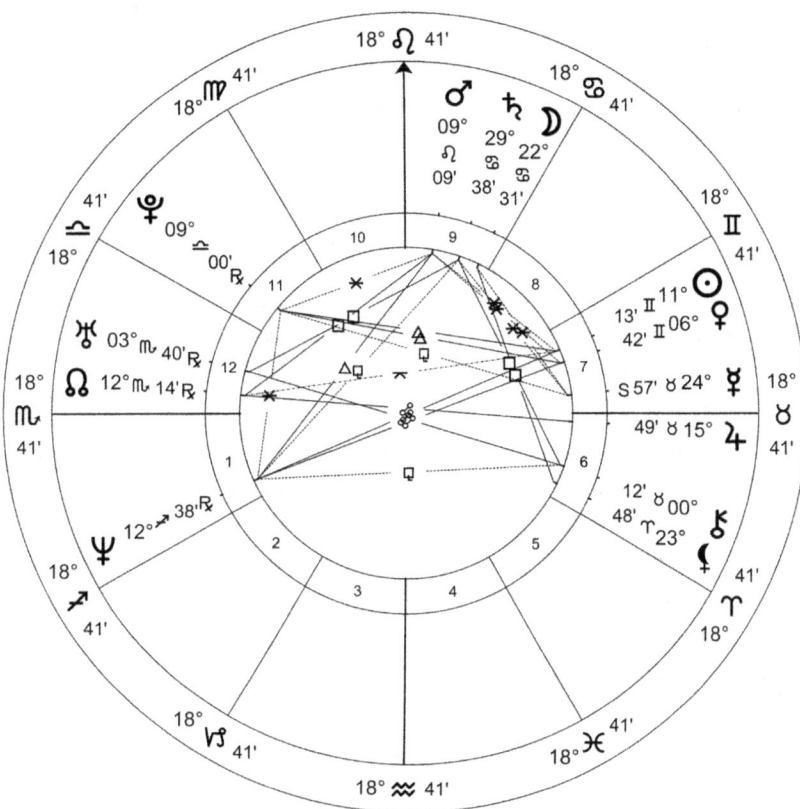

Figure 2. Patient's Chart.
Proserpina: 26 Libra 04; Pars of Disease: 11 Scorpio 36; Pars of Health: 14 Sagittarius 05

This sample Table of Dignities is quite unusual. It has a neutral planet: Saturn. As mentioned previously, transits may turn neutral planets in any direction. The other planets do not have high points, excluding two of them: the Hyleg and the Antihyleg. Both the Mercury Hyleg and Pluto Antihyleg have so-called absolute points. Points are considered absolute when there is only a plus or a minus. The planet with an absolute point acquires a lot of power, good or evil, depending on the result. In this case, Pluto as the Antihyleg with an absolute point evokes great apprehension, although Mercury Hyleg also has an absolute point and is a bit stronger than Antihyleg.

The person in question turned to me because he suffered unbearable headaches that traditional medicine could not ameliorate; no medication worked. It is precisely in these cases that people remember non-traditional medicine.

From a medical astrology perspective the illness seemed simple at first glance. It is very likely that a person with a T-square involving Mars and the lunar nodes would experience problems with his head, and of a karmic nature at that because of the influence of the nodes. There was also a Pole-axe pattern (square and two sesquiquadrates) with Neptune. Neptune is not a good planet according to the Tables of Dignities, and one could expect problems with the psyche. However, the Pars of Health was conjunct Neptune, and I did not observe any problems with the patient's psyche. There were quite powerful extrasensory abilities present in the patient, but ones he himself was afraid of and did not want to develop (this is not surprising with the Sun-Neptune opposition).

I asked the patient to request a head CT scan, just in case. He had already had some tests done, but they were inconclusive; however, they were not complete tests. Besides, I was alarmed by the approaching progressed square of Pluto and Mars. Having one as an Antihyleg and the other with a large degree of affliction (albeit with a positive status), one could expect anything, including a brain tumor. Moreover, in the chart these planets have an exact aspect, which, even though a sextile, still shows an initial energy connection between Pluto and Mars. Unfortunately the family physician declined the patient's request for the CT scan.

I performed energy healing for him and this brought him visible relief. However, he had to return again and again, as the source of the problem was not eliminated. A significant amount of spiritual work was also required of the patient. During the healing process it was important to draw attention to the Hyleg, as it was an exceptionally powerful planet, stronger than the Antihyleg. In this case the Hyleg was Mercury, so breathing techniques could help a lot.

Furthermore, in order to weaken the influence of the approaching negative progression, we used herbal therapy (see chapter fourteen).

Chapter Eight

Astrodiagnosis

The general rule of astrodiagnosis is: if the indicators involve the aspects and the Hyleg table (particularly the Antihyleg), the illness can occur on the organic, or cell, level. If the indicators involve only passive degrees and the Pars of Disease, the illness will only be on a functional level and will not spread to the organic. This is of course true if they are appropriately treated, or even better, prevented in advance.

If you are unfamiliar with some medical terms, you might find the medical glossary at the end of the book helpful.

Vision Disorders

Generally, two celestial bodies are responsible for sight: the Sun and Moon. Therefore, one must first take notice of whether the celestial bodies are afflicted. As well, Mercury has a definite relationship with sight. Several possible situations can be considered:

- One of the luminaries is the Antihyleg.
- The Pars of Disease is conjunction a nebula, as well as with one of the indicated planets (Sun, Moon, or Mercury).
- A nebula or a negative star is located in one of the passive degrees, afflicted by the celestial bodies, and the degree is pointing to sight.
- The Sun or the Moon is afflicted by negative aspects of the other planets near the lunar nodes (especially during a day of an eclipse).
- The Moon in a T-square with the lunar nodes brings shortsightedness. If the Sun is conjunct one of the nodes, the situation is aggravated.
- The above is true if the Sun is square the nodes and the Moon is conjunct one of the nodes.

The above-mentioned can be indicators of possible illness of the organs of sight. However, the situation can become significantly worse if during a waning Moon (as it is more conducive to eye illnesses) the Sun or Moon is located in the eighth house and also afflicted with aspects, conjunction with a nebula, or if in the degree of sight. Blindness can occur in this instance.

The influence of Uranus can be touched upon here. If the Sun or the Moon is in the degree of Uranus or in negative aspects to Uranus, it is an indicator of glaucoma (with the waning Moon) or a lesion of the optic nerve (with the waxing Moon).

If under the same conditions one were to switch Uranus with Saturn, then a cataract can result; if the same occurs with Mars, conjunctivitis can occur.

Chiron and Proserpina influence the separation of the cornea, especially if the Sun, the Moon, or Mercury is in the degree of Proserpina.

Night blindness is associated with Neptune.

Disorders of the Hearing Organs

Hearing is ruled by Saturn; therefore one must pay attention to its position. Located in the twelfth house, Saturn indicates weak hearing, especially if it is close to the Ascendant. Saturn in the sixth or twelfth house in conjunction with nebulas or malignant stars can bring serious hearing impairment. If Saturn is in negative aspect with the luminaries, the situation deteriorates. Here we are referring to congenital problems; however, there are also acquired hearing disorders as complications occurring after the underlying disease.

Saturn and the Moon will show whether complications associated with the ears will arise. Negative aspects between Saturn and the Moon complicate the situation. However, the main focus should still be on Saturn. Different scenarios are possible here: Saturn has a negative status and the Pars of Disease is located in one of Saturn's degrees; the Pars of Disease is in Aries in conjunction with Saturn; the Pars of Disease is in Aries and Saturn is in conjunction with a nebula. Many variations can be found, but all feature nebulas, Saturn, the Pars of Disease, and the degrees of hearing.

If Uranus is involved, then the acoustic nerve may be afflicted. For example, if the Pars of Disease is in the degree of Uranus conjunct Saturn.

If instead of Uranus the degrees of Mars or Pluto are considered along the same variation, then inflammation of the middle ear (otitis) can occur. Mars is always responsible for inflammatory processes.

Disorders of the Olfactory Organs

Strictly speaking, we only have one organ of smell: the nose. Diseases of the nose are quite complex as there are many planets involved. Jupiter and Uranus are involved in control over the faculty of smell, while Mars and Saturn control the nose. The two latter planets must be considered. Serious illnesses of the sinuses, such as sinusitis, sometimes lead to a weakening, or even loss, of smell.

As always, pay attention to the aspects and degrees, particularly to the correlation between Saturn and Jupiter. With a bad aspect of Saturn and Jupiter, or if Saturn is in the degree of Jupiter on an Ascendant in bad aspect, then there can be a host of ENT disorders. These composite illnesses will most likely manifest if Saturn, in conjunction with Jupiter, is in the sixth or twelfth house.

Disorders of the Taste Organs

As you may recall from the first chapter, Mars rules the sense of taste. As well, the sense of taste is directly related to Taurus (the throat and the tongue are connected to Taurus). Mars has to be in one of the critical degrees in negative aspects with Venus and the Moon for the sense of taste to become weaker or to disappear. Furthermore, Taurus and/or Pisces must be afflicted. Generally, taste disorders are complex and often arise as a complication from the principal underlying illness.

Disorders of the Skin and Somatosensory System

Here we pay attention to Venus and Jupiter, because Venus rules the sense of touch, and Jupiter rules the skin. As always, look at the aspects, degrees, and location in the houses, as well as the Pars of Disease and the existence of nebulas. The connections between Venus and Jupiter, even through degrees, are of great importance. For instance, Venus in the degree of Jupiter in the twelfth house, especially close to the Ascendant, can indicate skin conditions. Connections with nebulas vary. Not only is the connection important but also the negative aspects; these can be both active degrees (early signs of the disease) and passive degrees (the disease as a complication).

Other planets may also be involved with specific illnesses. For example, with *eczema* it could be Venus, Jupiter, and Mars. There may be different combinations: Jupiter as Antihyleg in the degree of Mars; Mars as Antihyleg with the Pars of Disease in the degree of Jupiter or Venus; The Pars of Disease in the degree of Mars with Jupiter, or Venus as the Antihyleg. With *psoriasis*, instead of Mars we study Uranus, again in varying combinations: Venus and Jupiter are the Antihyleg and the Pars of Disease is in the degree of Uranus, or Venus as the Antihyleg in connection with evil Uranus.

Study Mercury for *neurodermatitis*. An afflicted Gemini may also be involved here. For example, Venus or Jupiter as the Antihyleg in Gemini, or the Pars of Disease in Gemini.

Also note whether Capricorn is afflicted, as skin conditions are often related to disruptions in the metabolic processes. Do not forget that sometimes skin diseases reveal other more serious illness (for example, liver disease). By treating only the symptoms we drive the principal underlying illness further in, which of course does not make us healthier.

Illnesses of the Head

These illnesses are always associated with Mars as the ruler of Aries, which in turn is related to the head. An affliction in Aries, Capricorn, or Cancer is also of significance. Notice whether Mars is in the sixth or twelfth house, and if it has negative aspects. With a square of Mars and Saturn, the aftermath of injuries can manifest in headaches. In the non-medical horoscope, this same square will provoke these injuries.

Neuralgias, migraines, insomnias and overstrain are identified through the aspects between Mars and the Moon or through the position of Mars in the degree of the Moon. *Blood vessel spasms* and *nervous breakdowns* are also related to Uranus. To diagnose the above-indicated illnesses, one could look at various combinations: Mars as the Antihyleg afflicted by the Moon, or the Moon as the Antihyleg with a negative aspect from Mars; or if the Pars of Disease is with bad aspects from Mars or the Moon; evil Mars is in the degree of the Moon; and so on.

Although negative aspects or the connection between Mars and the Moon often predispose one to overstrain and insomnia, the positive aspects from the Sun (especially if the Sun is the Hyleg) compensate for this. The Sun brings enough life energy for the person to overcome the illnesses.

Diseases of the Respiratory System

Here we consider illnesses of the respiratory tract, lungs, and throat. Illnesses of the respiratory tract are always related to Mercury. The afflicted signs of Taurus, Gemini, Virgo, or Cancer are also involved here and the Pars of Disease in these signs can also play a role.

If we are examining the throat and tonsils, usually Venus is involved. Mercury in the degree of Venus in negative aspect, the Pars of Disease in the degree of Venus, Taurus on the Ascendant, and Mercury in a square with the Ascendant are all indicators of a weakened throat. If the bad influence of Mars is also present (Mercury is afflicted by Mars; the Ascendant is in the degree of Mars in Taurus), there is a possibility of inflammation of the tonsils, adenoids, and the nasopharynx in general. Loss of voice is also associated with Taurus, Mars, and Mercury.

Chronic bronchitis is connected with Mercury and the affliction of Gemini. Lunar nodes are also involved in the formation of the illness. For example, if one of the nodes (particularly the North node) is in the degree of Mercury and in negative aspect, predisposition to chronic bronchitis may occur.

Bronchial asthma is associated with Saturn and Mercury and afflicted Gemini. Negative aspects from the Moon only increase the probability of asthma.

Lung disease is predetermined by Mercury, as well as by its degrees and the Pars of Disease in a sign of Mercury (Gemini, Virgo). Moreover, Jupiter plays a definite role in the diagnosis of lung disease, especially when in negative aspect with Mercury. If there is acute *pneumonia*, look for the connection between Jupiter, Mercury, and Mars.

Predisposition to *tuberculosis* is associated with Neptune, Mercury, and Jupiter. Predisposition to *silicosis* (an occupational lung disease caused by the prolonged inhalation of crystalline silica dust, typically found among miners and foundry workers) is associated with the Moon, Proserpina, and Mars. *Pulmonary edema* is always associated with the Moon in a bad aspect with Mercury. With *emphysema*, one must look toward Mercury and Uranus with afflicted signs of Cancer and Pisces.

Cardio-vascular Diseases

The heart is ruled by the Sun. This is why the Sun in negative aspect, as well as the affliction of Leo or Aries, may bring about a predisposition to illnesses of the heart.

Bad aspects of the Sun, Mars, and Uranus, as well as affliction of Aries, bring a propensity for *heart attack*. *Angina* is brought on by Mars, the Sun, and eastern Saturn (ascending before the Sun) if Saturn is in conjunction with the Sun and in negative aspects with Mars. *Arrhythmia* is connected to the Sun, Uranus, and Mercury.

Leo on the Ascendant often brings *tachycardia*. It is also connected with Uranus; for example, if the Sun is in Aquarius (ruled by Uranus) and Uranus afflicts the Sun with a tense aspect. The situation is compounded if, in addition to this, Uranus or the Sun is the Antihyleg, or if the Pars of Disease is in Leo. Another example is evil Uranus on the Ascendant in negative aspect from an evil Sun.

Congenital heart defects are connected with the Sun, Mars, and Saturn, with the affliction from Leo or Aries.

While heart disease is determined mainly by the Sun, Uranus plays a major role in vascular disease. In order to determine if a predisposition to vascular diseases exists, we should look at how frequently Uranus occurs among negative indicators (Pars of Disease in the degree of Uranus or in Aquarius, an afflicted Uranus on the Ascendant, the Antihyleg in the degree of Uranus, and so on). If among all the mentioned indicators the Sun and Uranus form a negative aspect, this may give rise to a predisposition to *stroke*. If there is a T-square that includes Mars, Uranus, and the Sun, this is a serious indicator for stroke, possibly with paralysis.

Afflictions in Sagittarius, Aquarius, and Gemini are also included the diagnosis of vascular diseases.

Uranus also correlates to problems with *blood pressure*. An eastern Uranus above the horizon indicates high blood pressure (hypertension), while western Uranus below the horizon indicates low blood pressure (hypotension), although this is not always confirmed in practice. As previously stated, the position of Uranus brings only an initial predisposition. Thus a person with western Uranus below the horizon could in youth initially have the propensity toward hypotension, but then evolve toward hypertension.

Atherosclerosis is connected to Saturn, Uranus, and the Sun.

Diseases of the Gastro-intestinal Tract

Here we must consider various combinations of planets. Illnesses of the stomach are determined by the Moon and affliction in Cancer or Taurus. Adding negative aspects of Mars to this may denote a *gastric ulcer*. Mercury and the afflicted signs of Virgo and Capricorn point to disease of the intestines. If Mars is again involved in the aspects or through degrees, then *ulcerative colitis* may result. The duodenum is also influenced by Neptune.

Constipation is related to Scorpio (plus the influence of Saturn). Scorpio is also involved in the formation of *hemorrhoids* with the influence of afflicted Mars, the Moon, and Mercury.

As is generally known, illnesses of the stomach are often connected with changes in the acidity of gastric juices, whether increasing or decreasing. The predisposition to a certain level of acidity can be gauged by the position of Mars and the Moon relative to the Sun. With eastern Mars and western Moon, an increased level of acidity is seen in the majority of people. With the eastern Moon and western Mars, one could presume decreased acidity. Anacidity will be present in individuals who have both Mars and the Moon positioned in the same hemisphere relative to the Sun (either the eastern or the western).

Various inflammations of the abdominal cavity are connected to Mars and the lunar nodes. Mars, which is always related to acute processes, is also involved in the occurrence of *peritonitis*, along with an afflicted Virgo. *Appendicitis* is connected with Virgo and Jupiter.

Liver Diseases

Hepatitis is determined by Jupiter, the Moon, and Neptune in varying combinations. A propensity toward *cirrhosis* is driven by Jupiter, Venus, Mars, and Saturn (one of these must be the Antihyleg and in bad aspect with the other indicated planets).

Illnesses of the bile duct are associated with Jupiter and Saturn. If there are more indicators around Saturn, then gallbladder disease may be presupposed (such as gallstones).

Together, afflicted Jupiter, Saturn, and Mars may bring *cholecystitis*. If the Moon is also prominent in the chart, then the spleen also suffers. An afflicted Pisces would confirm this diagnosis.

Diseases of the Endocrine System

The endocrine system is connected with Venus and Neptune and partially with the Moon. Afflicted Cancer, Taurus, Scorpio, and Libra are also of importance.

Illnesses of the *pancreas* are determined by an afflicted Virgo. If in addition to this Mercury is in a bad aspect, *diabetes* may occur. Diabetes is a complex illness; Neptune must be present for it to occur and sometimes other planets as well.

Diseases of the *adrenal gland* are connected to Venus and Neptune. In illnesses of the *thyroid gland* Venus is the main planet, but often with the involvement of Neptune, Mercury, and afflicted Gemini and Taurus.

Illnesses of the reproductive system are connected to Scorpio, as well as Venus, Mars, and Neptune. If Pluto (ruler of Scorpio) is not in a good position, uterine or prostate cancer may occur.

Gynecological Diseases

These are connected with Mars, Venus, and the Moon.

Infertility is related to Mars, Venus, and especially Saturn in a bad aspect. If Saturn is also in the fifth house or its ruler, this greatly increases problems with childbirth. Infertility is also shown by the barren signs (Gemini, Virgo, and Aquarius) if the ruler of the fifth house is located in them.

The propensity toward *miscarriage* is connected to Scorpio, Taurus, and a strong element of water in the chart. However, Uranus in negative aspect is of particular significance here.

The Moon affects disorders of the menstrual cycle.

Diseases of the Skeletal System

Here we first deal with Saturn, although the afflicted signs of Capricorn, Aquarius, and Aries are also important. If Saturn is the Antihyleg in the horoscope, it is certain that there will be problems with the bones, spine, joints, and teeth.

Problems with the ligaments and cartilage are determined by Saturn and Mercury together.

The Sun, Mercury, and Uranus are connected to illnesses of the joints (arthritis, gout). Saturn, Mercury, and the Sun, as well as an afflicted Aquarius, are related to *rheumatism*. The brittleness of bones is connected with an affliction of Gemini.

Dental Diseases

Saturn and Mars exert the main influence here. The affliction of Aries and Capricorn is also important. Aries rules the head, while Capricorn rules the skeletal system in general. If the luminaries are afflicted by Saturn, or if Saturn is in its own degree with Mars as the Antihyleg, early tooth decay may result. Different combinations of Saturn and Mars, as well as the signs they rule, Aries and Capricorn, need to be viewed.

Gum disease can occur if Taurus is afflicted. Venus, Saturn, and Chiron in negative aspect would also need to be involved. Furthermore, the involvement of negative Mercury in this scenario is indicative of *periodontal disease*; for example, Saturn in the degree of Mercury and Mercury on the Ascendant, or Mercury and Saturn in conjunction, and so on.

Blood Diseases

Illnesses of the blood are very complex and cannot be determined by one or two planets; there must be a lot of evil planets active at once. These illnesses are mainly related to the Sun, Moon, Venus, and Jupiter. Saturn in a negative aspect can indicate a malfunction of blood-producing organs (bone marrow and spleen.) If there is a negative influence coming from Pluto, then cancer of the blood may occur. All forms of *leukemia* are directly related to Pluto.

Neptune and afflicted water signs are involved in the formation of *anemia*. The influence of Mars, which rules hemoglobin, is also probable.

Kidney Illnesses

The kidneys are ruled by Venus. *Kidney stones* are related to Venus and Saturn (Venus, kidneys;

Saturn, stones.) Capricorn is related to bladder illnesses.

Here are a few more illnesses of the urinary tract system: *nephritis*, Venus and the Moon; *uremia*, Mars with an afflicted Scorpio; *nephrosclerosis*, Venus, the Moon, Mars, and Saturn.

Diseases of the Nervous System

These diseases are connected with the Moon, Uranus, Neptune, and afflictions in water or air signs. Purely nervous illnesses (where emotions are more involved, but not the psyche as such) are determined by the Moon and Uranus. It is Neptune, first of all, and then the Moon and Uranus that are related to mental illness.

The Moon, Uranus, Neptune, and Saturn are related to *epilepsy*. *Paralyses* are connected with Saturn and Uranus. *Parkinson's disease* is determined by Saturn, Uranus, and Mercury.

Illnesses of the spinal cord are connected with Saturn and Uranus in equal measure. *Multiple sclerosis* may be brought on by bad aspects of Saturn, Uranus, and the Sun with an affliction in Capricorn, Aquarius, or Leo.

Mental Illnesses

First we look at the position of Neptune. *Schizophrenia* is connected with Neptune, Saturn, and the Moon. Uranus is not involved here. If Uranus is added, then *epilepsy* may result. Schizophrenia most often occurs among Pisces, Cancer, Capricorn, and Aries.

Paranoia is determined by Saturn, Neptune, the Moon, and Mars. Leo is most susceptible to paranoia.

Delirium and *alcoholic delusion* are related to Mars and Neptune. *Manic-depressive (Bipolar) disorder* is connected with the Sun, Moon, Saturn, and Neptune, with affliction of the air signs.

Chapter Nine

Reading a Medical Horoscope

You might feel uncomfortable after reading the previous chapter, having discovered the potential for one or more terrible illnesses in your horoscope—just as Jerome K. Jerome, upon reading a medical reference book, found he was suffering from every illness except for housemaid's knee.

You can relax, because the information in chapter eight alone is not sufficient to draw any conclusions. Even if there are strong indications of a certain disease, it makes sense to first look for favorable factors. For example, if the Sun and Moon are not afflicted, and are located in proximity to the angles (especially the Ascendant and Midheaven), and if the Hyleg is stronger than the Antihyleg, any potential illnesses may never come to pass. And even if you weren't very lucky, with the abovementioned indicators there is still no cause for worry as there are preventive measures available.

The following is the method I use to read a medical horoscope. You may want to modify this or create your own.

First evaluate the chart without the houses to easily reveal the simple illnesses for which the person has a predisposition. Look at the position of the planets in the signs, whether they are in fall or detriment. The aspects must also be considered. If there is a T-square, then the planets in its center are already weak. Finally, look at the signs.

There is a simple rule: if there is an accumulation of good planets in one of the signs (check the tables of dignities), then the organ or the system of the sign will be healthy. However, there is one "but" here: if the opposite sign does not have any planets, then the illnesses of that sign may appear. The sign will be initially weak, as the stellium of planets in the opposite sign will draw off energy. My daughter's horoscope serves as an example. She has a stellium in Scorpio, while Taurus is empty. As a result, she had congenital myogenic torticollis (wryneck), the neck being the part of the body ruled by Taurus. And in childhood she was afflicted with constant tonsillitis. Fortunately, illnesses of this sort usually pass with age.

If a stellium of evil planets is observed in a sign, then there is a great probability that illnesses characteristic of that sign will appear. In medical astrology the signs generally play a more significant role than houses, though there are exceptions: houses six, twelve, and four are important ones.

The status and position of the Hyleg and Antihyleg are more important than the parses and degrees. After analyzing the planets in the signs and the aspects we build the tables of dignities and locate the Hyleg and Antihyleg. It is important what kind of planets these are and where they are located. Only at the very end, as an addition, do we consider the Pars of Health and the Pars of Disease, and after that, if clarification is required, the degrees.

Always analyze houses six and twelve, generally as a pair. Those people who do not have planets in these houses are fortunate. If there are planets and they are evil, then the people are clearly burdened. Illnesses from the planets (and signs) located in houses six and twelve begin to appear first, even at an early age. This is especially true for the sixth house, as it brings an initial weakness to the planets. If Mars (or Aries) is in the sixth house, one can expect a person to suffer from headaches or hemorrhoids at a rather early age. If Saturn is present, problems with the skeletal system are likely to occur, such as juvenile scoliosis. Planets in the twelfth house are not as pronounced; they mainly manifest on the psychosomatic level.

The fourth house is checked for genetic diseases. However, if the planet located in the fourth house is good and does not have negative aspects, one could suppose that there will be no negative genetic dispositions for the person.

The positions of the planets in houses one and ten are considered favorable.

Patient with Headaches

We'll use the chart (Figure 2) from chapter seven as an example of interpretation of the medical horoscope. The person came to me because of terrible headaches that traditional medicine could not successfully treat, nor even find the cause.

A first glance at the natal chart draws attention to Mars in the center of a T-square involving the lunar Nodes and Jupiter. The presence of the nodes brings a tinge of inevitability to the picture. The position of Mars could of course indicate migraines. However, it's not that simple. Let's take a look at the medical status of the planets.

Su	Mo	Mer	Ven	Mar	Jup	Sat	Ura	Nep	Plu	Pro	Chi
+8	+7	+12	+7	+6	+9	+7	+2	+4	0	+4	+14
-6	-11	0	-13	0	-6 -5	-7	-5	-7	-9	-3	-13
+2	-4	+12a	-6	+6a	-2	0	-3	-3	-9a	+1	+1

It is evident from the table that the majority of this patient's planets have a neutral status. Mercury the Hyleg, Pluto the Antihyleg, and Venus stand somewhat apart. Both the Hyleg and the Antihyleg have an absolute point, which makes them even stronger. Pluto does not have a single serious negative aspect and is located in the neutral eleventh house. A fleeting glance at the horoscope would not cause anyone to pay attention to Pluto. However, an absolute point of "-9" is cause for concern.

In addition, progressed Pluto was approaching a square with Mars, which altogether did not occasion optimism. Pluto and Mars are the rulers of the Ascendant and the Pars of Disease. Transiting Saturn was conjunct Mars at about the same time. In terms of energy treatments, I did what I could. I also insisted that my patient visit his family doctor in order to obtain a medical referral for a head scan in order to exclude the presence of a tumor. Unfortunately, the doctor declined to issue the referral, deciding that there were insufficient grounds. In this case I also recommended herbs for the prevention of possible complications. I used a Venus plant to mitigate the power of Mars and Pluto (see chapter fourteen).

Knowing which planet is the Hyleg we can use its power to increase the energy of the organism and, as a result, its recovery. In this case Mercury is the Hyleg. All types of breathing practices were very effective to the recovery of this particular individual.

Jupiter and Chiron are in the sixth house. Jupiter is conjunct the South Node, which weakens its power. According to the tables of dignities, Jupiter is almost neutral (a slightly negative point). Despite this, Jupiter did not cause me concern. Besides, the Pars of Health is in Sagittarius, the sign of Jupiter.

Uranus, Proserpina, and the Pars of Disease are located in the twelfth house. However, the position of the planets in the twelfth house does not yet indicate the presence of disease. In this case it is unlikely to bring the patient any problems: only slight blood pressure surges. What needs to be tracked here is the sign in which the Pars of Disease is located. With time, Scorpio can bring problems with the sexual sphere, the more so since Pluto, ruler of Scorpio, is the Antihyleg.

Saturn and the Moon are located in the center of a T-square. The Moon has a negative point, while Saturn is neutral. Problems with bones and the stomach are possible but not absolute. Problems with the gastrointestinal tract may arise if one was to worry a lot or not adhere to a suitable diet.

What looks much more problematic is Neptune. It is located in the center of the pole-axe configuration (two aspects with 135 degrees plus a square) in the first house. The pole-axe is powerfully manifested in psychosomatic illnesses. Furthermore, Neptune is in opposition to the Sun and Venus. The sufficient quantity of the water element in the chart and the position of the Moon in Cancer, as well as all the above-mentioned indicators, show a strong nervous excitability of the patient. The nervous system is very sensitive, although the likelihood of serious disorders is not strong because Neptune is conjunct the Pars of Health, somewhat improving its status.

With the negative status of Venus and Neptune, and the opposition between them, it makes sense to check the working of the pancreas in order not to miss symptoms of diabetes. Diabetes is not a genetic illness in this case. The empty fourth house reveals the absence of illnesses transmitted by genetics.

Chronic Illness

Now let's consider another natal chart (Figure 3). What immediately jumps out is Saturn in Capricorn in the sixth house, the house that indicates how an illness will progress. In this case it is in Capricorn; therefore, one could presuppose a tendency to chronic illnesses. This woman suffers from several chronic illnesses, although acute conditions rarely happen. If Aries is in the sixth house, illnesses in general are acute but pass quickly.

The presence of Saturn in the sixth house also testifies to an early diagnosis of skeletal system disorders. In her teenage years the patient was diagnosed with scoliosis and later with osteochondrosis. Problems with the spine and joints have attended this individual throughout her life. The fact that Saturn is the Antihyleg clearly "helps" this, as does the Pars of Disease, which is located in Capricorn.

In the twelfth house we see Mercury, which raises the question of respiratory system illnesses of a psychosomatic nature. However, the status of Mercury as the Hyleg with an absolute positive point plays a more important role than its presence in the twelfth house. With the exception of a couple cases of childhood pneumonia, diseases of the lungs or bronchi were not observed.

The Ascendant is in Leo; however, this does not in itself indicate heart problems. (Some Sun-sign books foretell illness based on the Sun-sign alone, but it is more complicated than that. So, if you are a Cancer, you will not necessarily have a weak stomach; if you are a Scorpio, you will not necessarily have problems within the sexual sphere; and so on.)

Su	Mo	Mer	Ven	Mar	Jup	Sat	Ura	Nep	Plu	Pro	Chi
+4	+6	+13	0	+4	+10	+9	+7	+4	+6	+8	+4
0	-10	-3	-6	-11	-7	-16	-7	0	-10	0	-4
+4a	-4	+10	-6a	-7	+3	-7	0	+4a	-4	+8a	0

This person has two Antihylegs with the same number of points in her horoscope: Saturn and Mars. The Hyleg is Mercury; Venus is strongly negative and the Moon is slightly negative. Proserpina is extremely positive, with an absolute number of positive points. Neptune is also positive. The Sun and Jupiter are moderately good. The other planets are more or less neutral.

Mars, as the second Antihyleg, also revealed itself, though only at a later age, bringing hemorrhoids (but again, in a more chronic rather than acute form) and problems with the sexual sphere in the form of uterine fibroids. Uterine fibroids, although initially very small, provoked very heavy bleeding and in turn led to chronic anemia. You may recall that Mars is responsible for hemoglobin. Problems with the female sexual organs were genetic: Scorpio in the fourth house as well as Neptune in the fourth house opposition Mars.

Neptune does not indicate mental disorders because it is not in the genetics and Neptune itself is good. However, Neptune is located in the center of a highly unpleasant "pole-axe" configuration, which indicated repeated depression. The Moon was also involved.

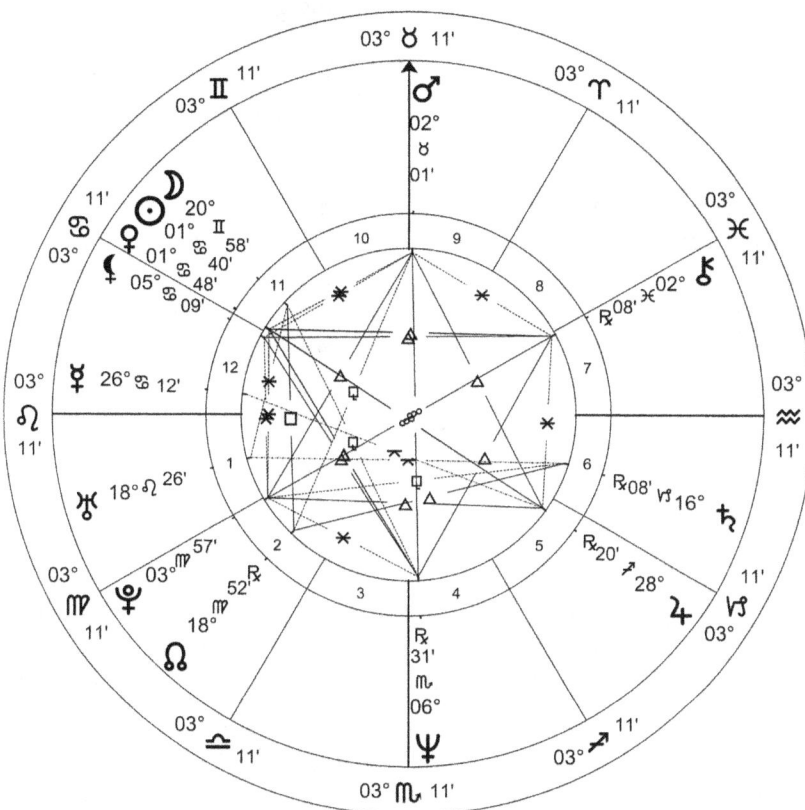

Figure 3. Patient's Chart.
Proserpina: 18 Libra 37; Pars of Disease: 8 Capricorn 01; Pars of Health: 6 Aquarius 31

Note that the Moon is positioned in the center of a T-square, indicating a sensitive nervous system. The Moon did not indicate stomach problems, but it did reflect poor eyesight. Illnesses do not always pass across the spectrum of the planets. The individual developed early shortsightedness, and later astigmatism. But one of the patient's eyes was always better than the other, which is not surprising if it's taken into account that one of the eyes is ruled by the Moon and the other by Proserpina.

Venus is not combust, but it is a cazimi (within seven minutes of an exact conjunction with the Sun). Venus has a fairly strong negative point. The woman did not have kidney problems, but did have an early diagnosis of thyroid gland illness. And Venus began to negatively influence the Sun, "eating" it from the inside. Dysfunction of the thyroid provoked constant tachycardia, although heart disease was not "prescribed" in the chart.

The two Antihylegs brought one more illness. Saturn and Mars rule the nose, and this person had perpetual nasal congestion for twenty-five years. The nasal congestion was of an allergic nature, which was finally overcome with a three-year course of allergy shots.

At age thirty the woman also developed a rather complicated illness: eczema; Venus, Mars, and Jupiter are associated with eczema. Mars Antihyleg is located in the degree of Jupiter. Jupiter is fairly positive, but is opposition Venus. The South Moon Node is located in the degree of eczema and skin allergies.

One should also remember to take notice of the degrees, even though they are secondary indicators. The woman's Saturn, the Antihyleg, is located in the degree of the endocrine system and, as discussed above, the endocrine system is definitely not in order. Uranus is in the degree of predisposition to hypertension; this planet rules the circulatory system. On its own, Uranus is neutral without negative aspects; also, the Pars of Health is located in Aquarius. However, hypertension still arose, but only in later years and in a weak form.

Unfortunately, Mercury, the Hyleg in this chart, is an isolated planet; it does not have a single major aspect. Therefore, its part in the harmonization of health is limited, as it's difficult for it to influence other planets.

Autistic Child

Figure 4 is the chart of an autistic child. Although autism is generally considered an illness, I believe it more likely that it is a state of the mind and soul. Some Indigo children have autistic symptoms. Neptune, Saturn, and the Moon are the main planets associated with this condition.

In the majority of cases people experiencing problems in communication with others have important planets in the twelfth house. In this example the Sun and Mercury (responsible for communication) are located in the twelfth house (in both the Placidus and Medical systems). Mercury is opposition Pluto, which adds complications with socializing in groups. Neptune and Saturn form an opposition. The Moon is in a T-square with Jupiter and the lunar nodes; the nodes add a karmic influence. All these indications show possible problems in social behavior but not necessarily an illness. This child is very kind and a joy in his mother's life.

Having determined which illnesses may appear and which are unlikely to do so, in the next chapter we'll look at predicting the time when they may occur.

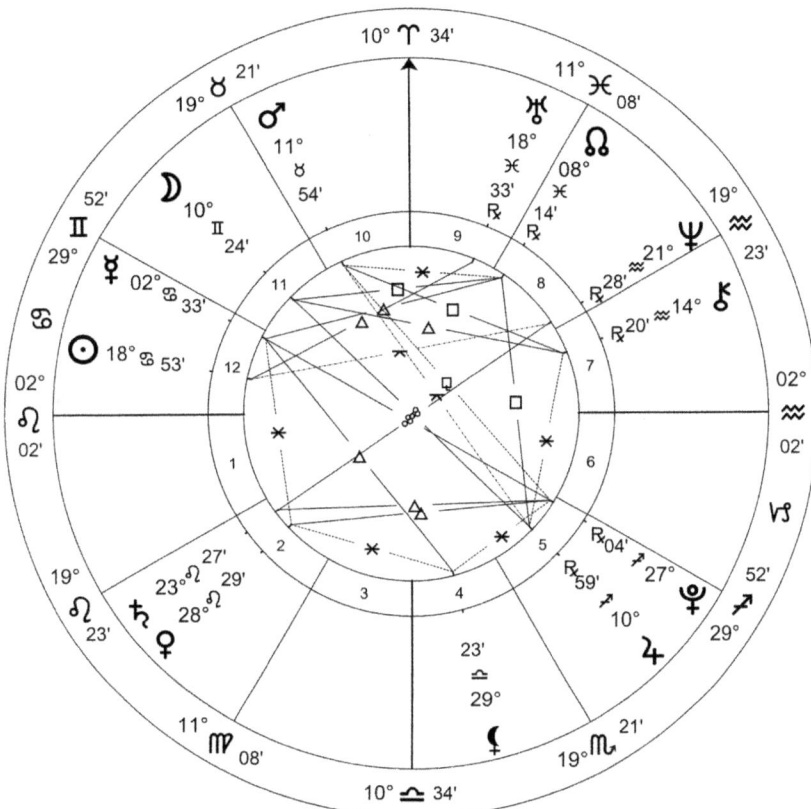

Figure 4. Patient's Chart.

Chapter Ten

Predicting the Timing of Illness

As has been previously mentioned, the indication of weak organs and systems in the chart doesn't mean an inevitability of disease. A trigger is needed for the beginning of illness and this greatly depends on planetary influences. As a rule, ailments connected to the signs of the Ascendant and sixth house show themselves early (if those illnesses are indicated). Transits, progressions, and symbolic rhythms are used for forecasting the time when the health impairment can be expected.

Symbolic Planetary Rhythms

The planetary age periods can be significant and each is ruled by a specific planet:

- 0-7 years: Moon
- 7-14 years: Mercury
- 14-23 years: Venus
- 23-36 years: Sun
- 36-46 years: Mars
- 46-63 years: Jupiter
- 63-84 years: Saturn
- 84 plus years: Uranus

Other planets don't participate because we are unlikely to live long enough to reach the age at which their influence begins.

You might find the age period of your Antihyleg and wonder whether you'll be ill for all those years. Don't worry; you won't. Antihyleg may show significant influence for the age period only if it is located in an angular house. If it is in the cadent house it is almost invisible in this regard.

However, Antihyleg certainly influences the state of health in the year it rules. This is true also for Hyleg and other strong planets.

Symbolic cycles of years of life and their are defined as follows:

Year of Life	Ruled by
First	Mars
Second	Sun
Third	Venus
Fourth	Mercury
Fifth	Moon
Sixth	Saturn
Seventh	Jupiter
Eighth	Pluto
Ninth	Sun
Tenth	Neptune
Eleventh	Uranus
Twelfth	Moon
Thirteenth	Saturn and Proserpina
Fourteenth	Jupiter and Chiron

The sequence then repeats from the beginning. For example, the fifteenth year is ruled by Mars, the sixteenth by the Sun, the seventeenth by Venus, and so on.

In the years of malicious planets, health can be greatly impaired. Any negative transits are strongly felt, although they might be almost invisible in the years of favorable planets. For example, if a person has malicious Moon, Saturn, and Jupiter, the period from forty-six to forty-eight years (the years ruled by these planets) might be remembered as a time when diseases followed one another. The illnesses, however, might not be related to the ruling planet. The organism is simply weakened in these years and has a low resistance to ailments. Specific problems are determined by transiting planets.

Years of Antihyleg in the age period of Antihyleg are especially unpleasant. For instance, for Mars Antihyleg, the chance for a serious illness is significant at age forty-two (forty-third year). If, however, Mars is Hyleg, then at age forty-two one's health can be expected to be excellent. Although the organism doesn't care about transit squares, a T-square or a grand cross could be influential. Even in this case the recovery will be fast.

Throughout our lifetime we experience the influence of a huge number of transits and progressions. In order not to get confused we need to learn to distinguish which of them are important and which are not. For recognition of significant transits we need symbolic rhythms. However, progressions and transits will always represent the most important indications of the beginning of possible diseases.

Transits and Progressions in Medical Astrology

In medical astrology I use symbolic progressions: one degree equals one year. Secondary progressions could also be effective, but I have not used them in medical astrology except with midpoints.

The rules of diagnostics described below can be used for transit situations as well. The rule here is the same as in general predictive astrology: one can experience only those situations that were written in one's natal chart. If a planet is affected by negative transits and there is a confirmation in the natal chart, we can assume the onset of illness. The planets will show what kind of illness is most likely. For example, the affliction of Jupiter in the year of "evil" Jupiter might bring liver disease. If Neptune, in a bad year, afflicts the Moon, it could bring poisoning with hard consequences for the gastro-intestinal tract. If there is also a Mars influence, consequences are guaranteed.

However, if this transit happened in a good year and Neptune and especially the Moon are not malicious, then only light poisoning without consequences could occur (or not happen at all). It is always necessary to remember that transits and progressions work not only on the medical level but also on the level of events. Usually it is one or the other and only rarely on both levels. Thus, with the absence of the particular illness confirmation in the natal chart, negative transits may provoke only mild un-wellness that is usually effectively treated by traditional medicine.

For determination as to what organs may be affected we also need to take into consideration signs and degrees. It is not always true that the organ of a planet to which the power of the aspect is directed will become ill. For example, if Saturn makes a square or opposition to the Sun it doesn't mean the certainty of heart disease. General weakening of health might be expected, thereby allowing all chronic illnesses to become more acute.

Diagnosis of cancer is the trickiest one. Cancer is almost always related to Pluto, and so far I've seen only one exception (see below). Oncological diseases may stay in a latent phase for a very long period during which it is difficult to detect them. They might appear at a bad aspect of Pluto but not be visible in the beginning. Early diagnosis is more probable if Pluto is strong and located in the sixth or twelfth house. If in the years of malicious Pluto a T-square or a grand cross is formed around Antihyleg, Hyleg, or Pluto, this can be the beginning of cancer even though it might not be diagnosed at once.

Brain Tumor

The chart in Figure 5 belongs to a man diagnosed with a brain tumor in November 2006. At this time progressed Pluto made a square to Mars in the twelfth house in Cancer, the sign of its fall. This is a classic example because the tumor "settled down" in the brain, which is ruled by Mars. The exact aspect took place earlier, in the spring of 2006, allowing the cancer to remain in a latent phase for several months and only later showing itself. It can actually be in a hidden stage much

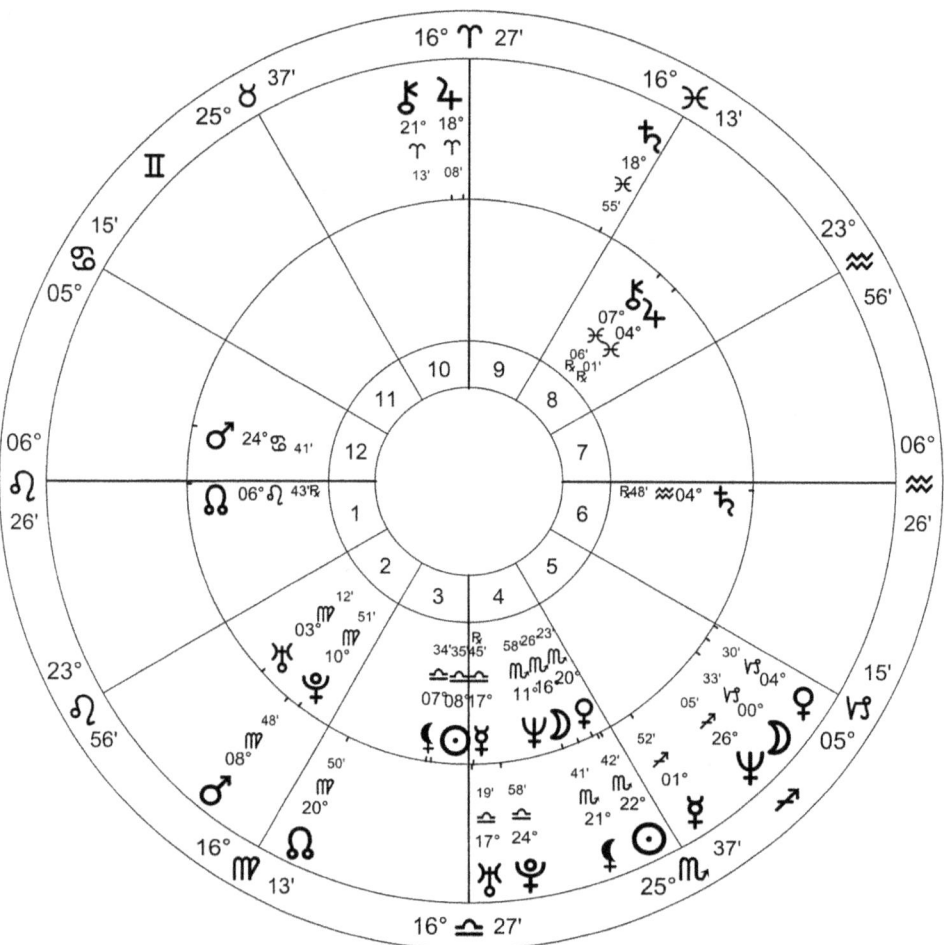

Figure 5. Inner Wheel: Natal Chart; Outer Wheel, Directed Progressions

longer. In this case, if the disease didn't become apparent in 2006, it would have been discovered at the end of 2008, when Pluto and progressed Mars were conjunct.

Transits also prove that the illness stayed in a latent phase for a while (Figure 6). The opposition of transiting Uranus to Pluto is especially prominent here; however, this transit is not enough to indicate the beginning of disease; it was triggered by both transits and progressions. Uranus formed the opposition a few times as it traveled retrograde and direct, the first time coming close in June 2005 (it turned retrograde six minutes before exactitude). Nothing happened at that time. Then Uranus repeated the opposition to Pluto in March 2006, which coincided with the progressions; this was the beginning of the illness. Then Uranus repeated the aspect in November 2006, and turned direct in opposition to Pluto (within minutes of exactitude); this was when the tumor was diagnosed.

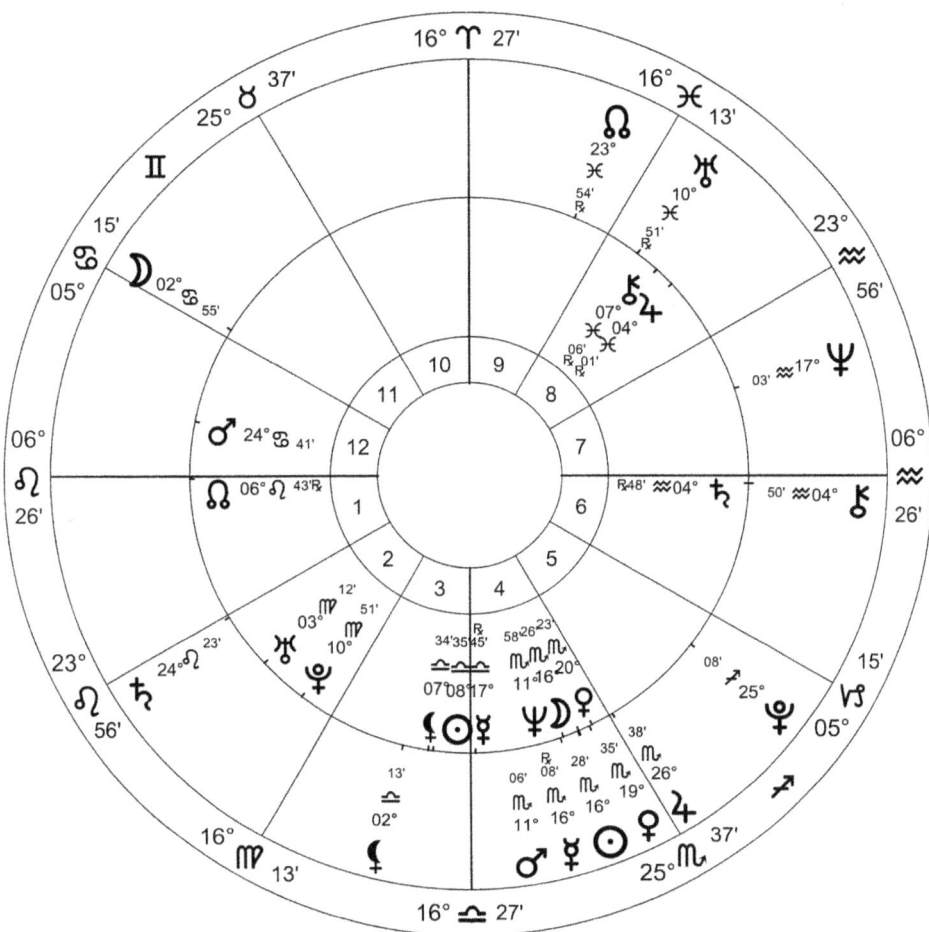

Figure 6. Inner Wheel: Natal Chart; Outer Wheel, Transits

Lymphoma

Only in one case in my practice was cancer not directly related to Pluto; in that case it was Proserpina. Proserpina plays a major role in AIDS and, in general, illnesses related to mutation. If we consider that cancer is in general a mutation, then the importance of Proserpina is understandable. Figure 7 is the chart of a girl who developed cancer at age sixteen. In this case I used Placidus houses because the chart is more demonstrative. In this chart Pluto is opposition the Sun, but Proserpina is in the center of a T-square with Jupiter and Saturn. Both Pluto and Proserpina are located in the eighth house.

At the time the illness was diagnosed, progressive Proserpina was conjunct Pluto (Figure 8). Progressed Black Moon (Lilith) was conjunct Neptune and opposition Mars. The role of Lilith in this

Medical Astrology for Healing

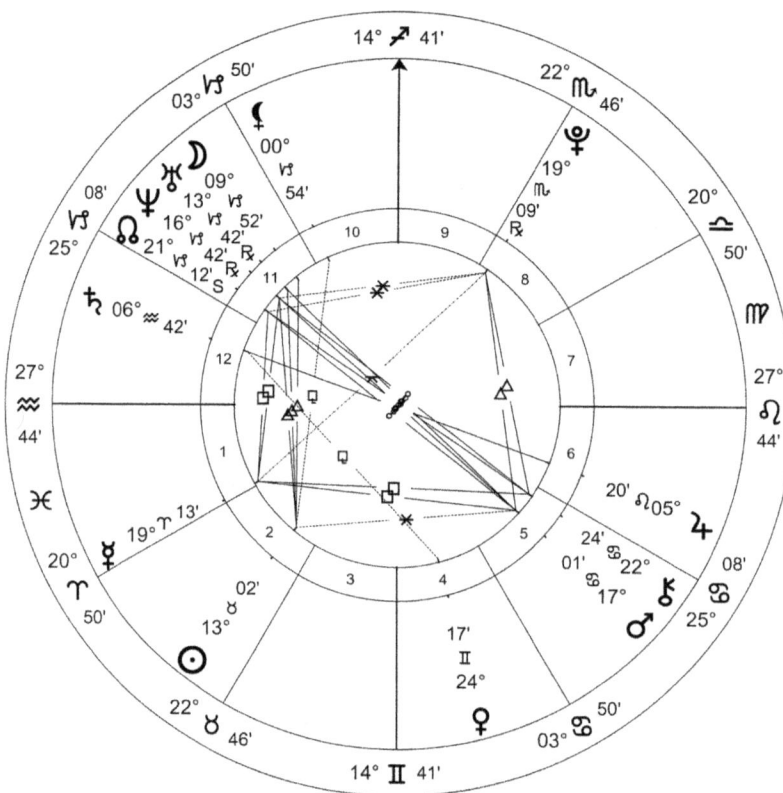

Figure 7. Patient's Chart. Proserpina: 3 Scorpio 15

particular case was significant because a manipulation from the black magic side acted as a trigger for the beginning of the disease. Progressed Mars formed a square to Proserpina, which also received an opposition from progressed Mercury. In addition to all of that, transiting Saturn from the sixth house formed a square to Pluto in the eighth house. The girl had one of the most complicated forms of cancer: lymphoma, with a lot of "knots" in the upper part of the body.

The girl's mother came to me after two years of visiting hospitals. The daughter had undergone surgery and chemotherapy with no improvement. Application of some non-traditional methods brought quick and sufficient improvement: the girl was able to live a normal life. However, the disease hadn't left forever. I knew that two years later the patient would face a dangerous time.

At the end of 2010 and beginning of 2011, transiting Proserpina formed an opposition to the natal Sun; the entire development of this illness was based on Proserpina rhythms. Simultaneously, progressed Mars from the sixth house made an opposition to Saturn in the twelfth house (Figure 8). Progressed Saturn was passing the Ascendant. Progressed Uranus, which rules Ascendant, formed

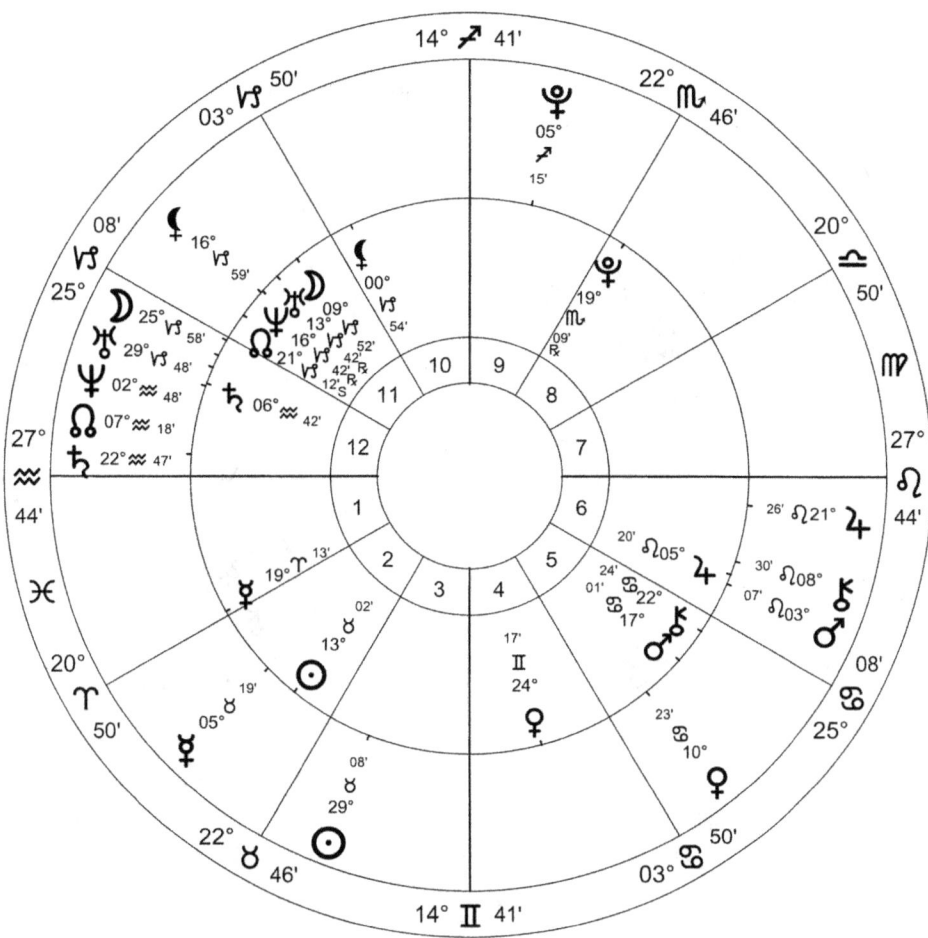

Figure 8. Beginning of the Disease.
Inner Wheel: Natal Chart; Outer Wheel, Directed Progressions
Progressed Proserpina: 19 Scorpio 20

a square to Proserpina. Unfortunately, the forecast in this case was not positive, and the situation suddenly worsened. (See Figure 9 on the next page.)

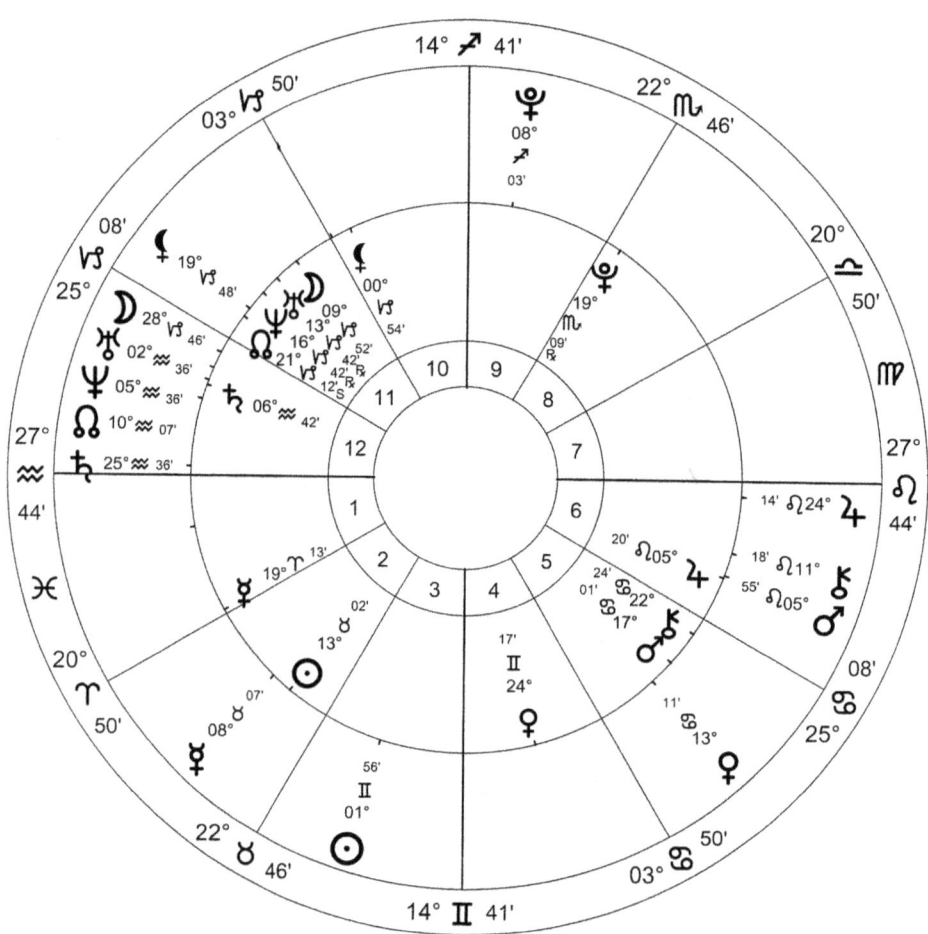

Figure 9. Progressions 2010.
Inner Wheel: Natal Chart; Outer Wheel, Directed Progressions
Progressed Proserpina: 22 Scorpio 55

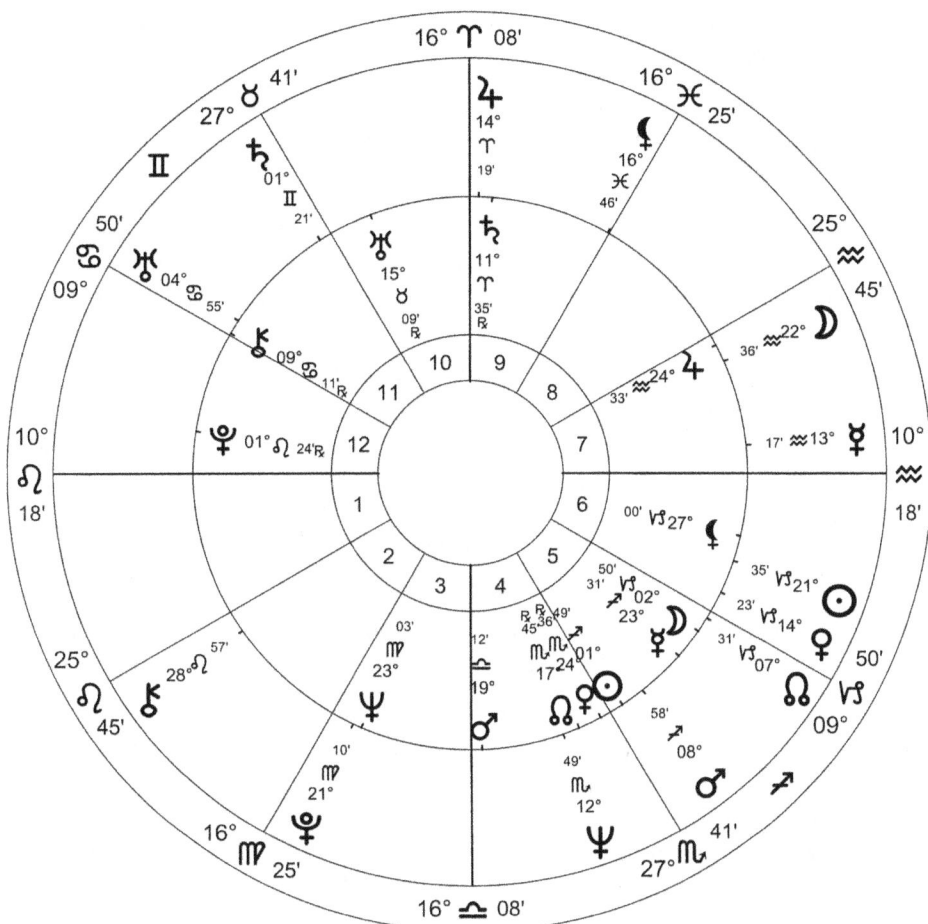

Figure 10. Disease Manifestation.
Inner Wheel: Natal Chart; Outer Wheel, Directed Progressions

Uterine Cancer

The woman whose chart is shown in Figure 10 was taken to the hospital by ambulance with severe bleeding. Uterine cancer was diagnosed and surgery and radiotherapy followed. There were no metastases and no relapses during the following twenty years.

The trigger was the opposition of progressed Saturn to natal Sun. The woman has a Leo Ascendant in Placidus (Cancer in the medical system), which is why the Sun has an important role. There are no indications in the horoscope for heart problems. As I mentioned before, the illness is not always related to the planet impacted by the negative aspect. Here Saturn could trigger any kind of disease, especially because it rules the sixth house. I pay even more attention to progressions than to transits because their influence lasts longer and lays serious cycles. Using the Placidus chart, Saturn rules the sixth house (health), and the Sun rules the first house (personality), and with an opposition like this, serious health problems can be expected.

Transits were active as well: retrograde Mars was aspecting Saturn and formed a square to the cusps of the sixth and twelfth houses. Because of this the woman remained in the hospital for four months.

At first, Pluto doesn't evoke any apprehensionp; it is in the first medical house and trine the Sun. However, if we dig deeper we discover that Pluto is the Antihyleg (together with Uranus) with a very high absolute point (-16). A positive aspect between Pluto and the Sun, though, played a role in final recovery.

But when did this cancer start? How long did the latent phase last? Probably not long, i.e., the tumor didn't produce metastasis. The only indication I found of the beginning of the process was a square from transiting Proserpina to Pluto a year and a half before the acute manifestation of disease.

Injury

I give a great deal of attention to oncological diseases because they are among the most complicated and, if found early in the latent phase, much can be done for their amelioration (if they are not karmic). With the help of energy and herbal healing it is possible to stop cancer at its onset.

Injuries are the most primitive from the astrological viewpoint. However, they are not the simplest in consequences. Figure 11 is an example of a transit situation for the moment of the injury: the fracture of an ankle bone. Transiting Mars was in a T-square with the lunar nodes. In addition, the progressed planets show a conjunction of Mars and Saturn. Having those two indicators is more than enough. It makes sense also to check the patient's chart to see if there is any chance for a broken bone. Saturn has a difficult square to Uranus, and fractures are almost always related to Saturn because it rules the skeletal system. Having Mars alone isn't enough. Mars more often brings bruises, cuts, burns, and surgery. The mentioned T-square makes the situation worse, indicating karma and inevitability. Both my surgeries happened on the same T-square with Mars and the lunar nodes: transiting in one case and progressed in the other one. I knew then that it was inevitable.

I haven't seen a lot of cases with other illnesses in my practice, which is not surprising as few people would go to an astrologer or healer with non-serious problems like cold or flu. With some other diseases it is almost impossible to find their beginning. This is why it is so difficult to construct a horoscope for a disease, known as a decumbiture (see chapter eleven).

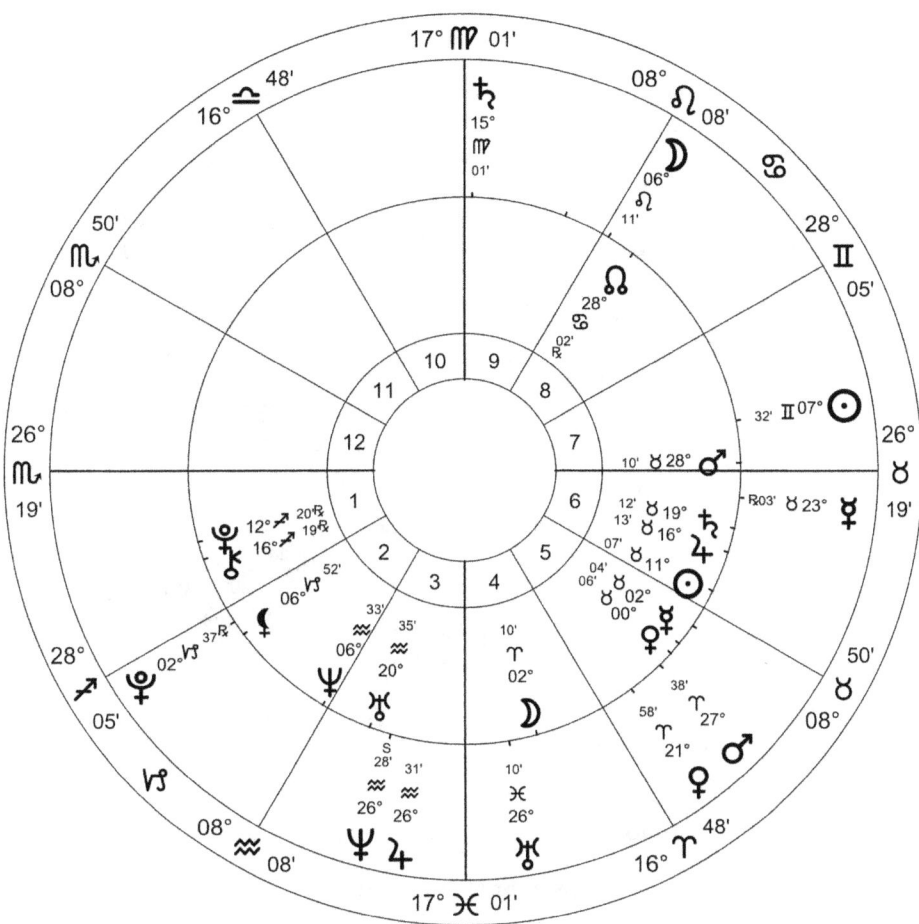

Figure 11. Bone Fracture
Inner Wheel: Natal Chart; Outer Wheel, Transits

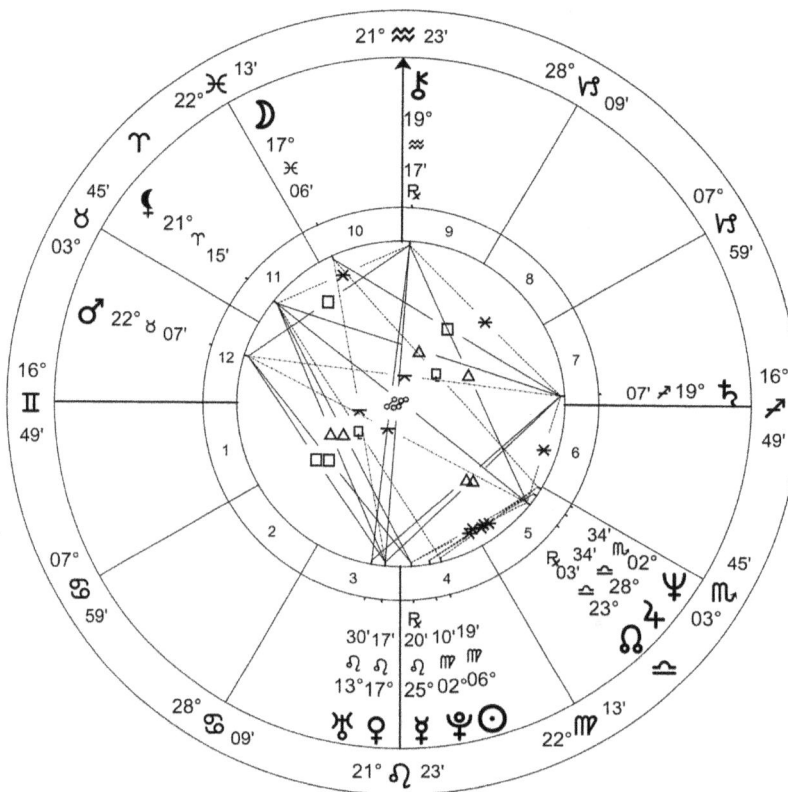

Figure 12. Michael Jackson Natal Chart.

Michael Jackson

Some cases are odd, such as the sudden death of Michael Jackson. Given a look at his natal chart I couldn't see any indications for heart attack (which was named as the cause of death in the beginning). One thought didn't leave me: "something was wrong with his medications"; however, there was no proof for this on the surface.

It is difficult to construct a chart for Michael Jackson because information about his birth time is conflicting, ranging from morning until late evening. It isn't surprising considering there were nine children in the family. I decided to choose 11:53 p.m. (Figure 12), which gives Gemini as the rising sign. Considering his appearance, Michael clearly had an air sign rising (particularly Aquarius or Gemini).

In this case the time of birth was not so important; aspects were more significant, or rather the lack of them as (Figure 13) as there were no serious progressions or transits.

There were no aspects concerning the Sun (heart). There was only one worth considering: an op-

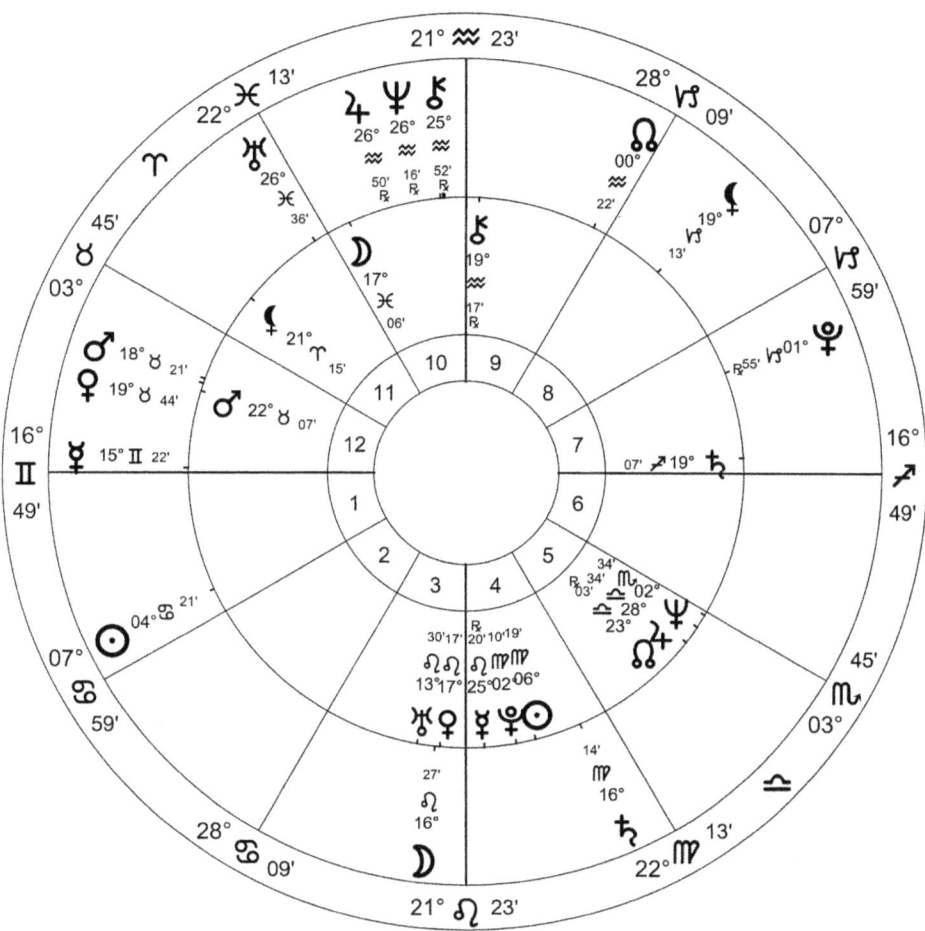

Figure 13. Michael Jackson Death
Inner Wheel: Natal Chart; Outer Wheel, Transits

position of transiting Neptune to natal Mercury. Neptune rules medications (affecting the nervous system, especially), drugs, and poison. Mercury rules the respiratory system. There is an impression that the person took medication and then stopped breathing. It probably wouldn't be so bad if Mercury weren't the ruler of Ascendant.

Medical Astrology for Healing

83

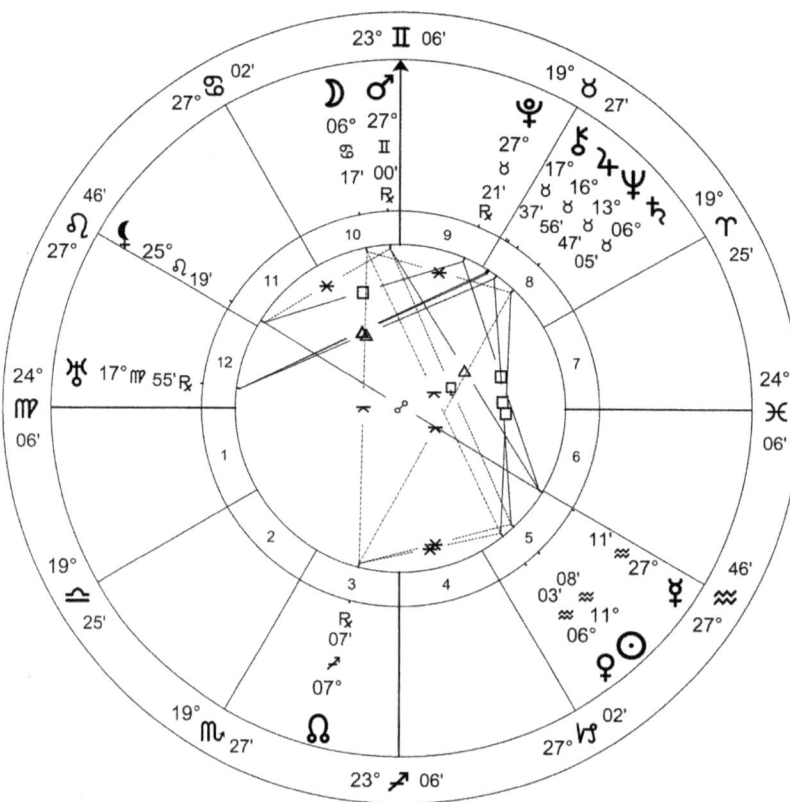

Figure 14. Franklin Roosevelt Natal Chart.

Poliomyelitis

Poliomyelitis can result in terrible health consequences, as well as for life in general. As an example, look at the chart of Franklin Delano Roosevelt, former president of the United States (Figure 14).

In August 1921, Roosevelt became very sick, and poliomyelitis was diagnosed. He suffered a partial paralysis and was never again able to walk freely. Physicians later determined that this was not exactly polio but Guillain-Barré syndrome. However, the exact diagnosis isn't important in determining the astrological conclusions.

The trigger in this case was Neptune. Neptune always has a connection to all unusual diseases when the diagnosis is unclear. Polio is an infectious disease, but it affects mostly the nervous system, which is ruled by Neptune.

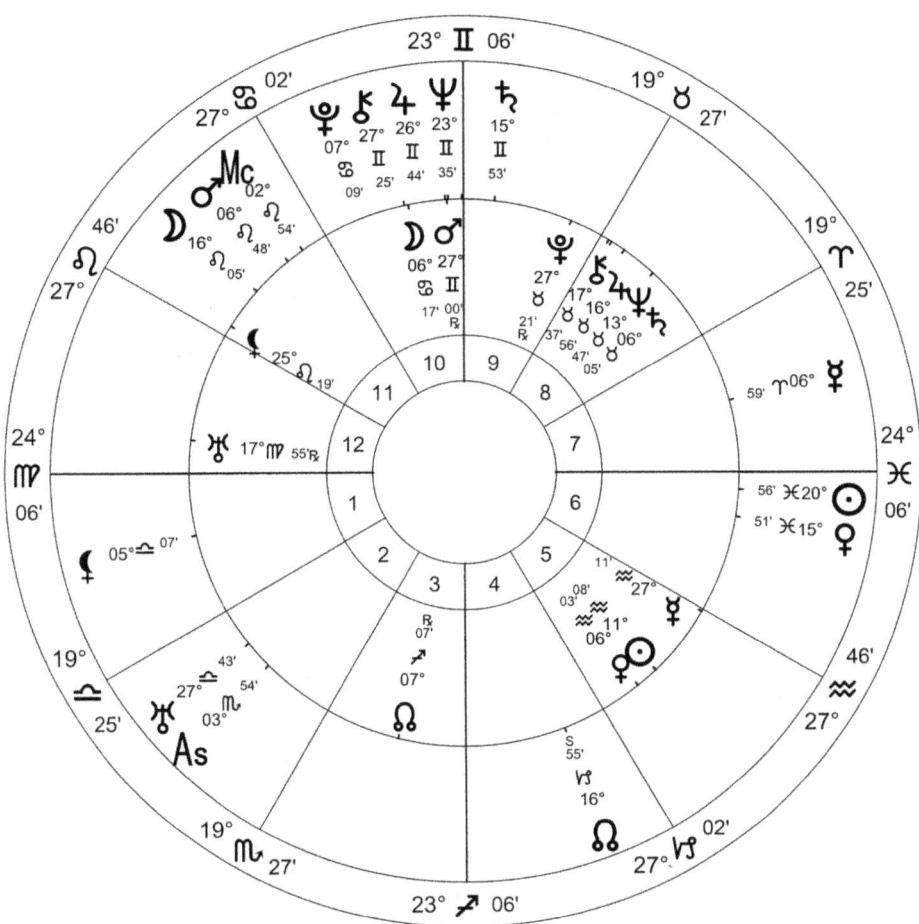

Figure 15. Franklin Roosevelt
Inner Wheel: Natal Chart; Outer Wheel, Directed Progressions
Progressed Proserpina: 22 Libra 44

In the progressed chart for the beginning of the illness (Figure 15), Neptune is square the Ascendant (Placidus cusps). In addition to Neptune, the cusp of the eighth house reaches Pluto, and cusps of the sixth and twelfth houses form a T-square with the Moon.

Neptune in transit is even more impressive (Figure 16). First, it makes a square to itself. Second, Black Moon (Lilith) also forms a square to Neptune. Thus, natal Neptune finds itself in the center of a T-square with transiting Neptune and Black Moon. Neptune in this chart is in the eighth house (extreme circumstances). The presence of Lilith shows the connection to karmic debts. Transiting Mars forming a T-square with Saturn and Venus was the final trigger.

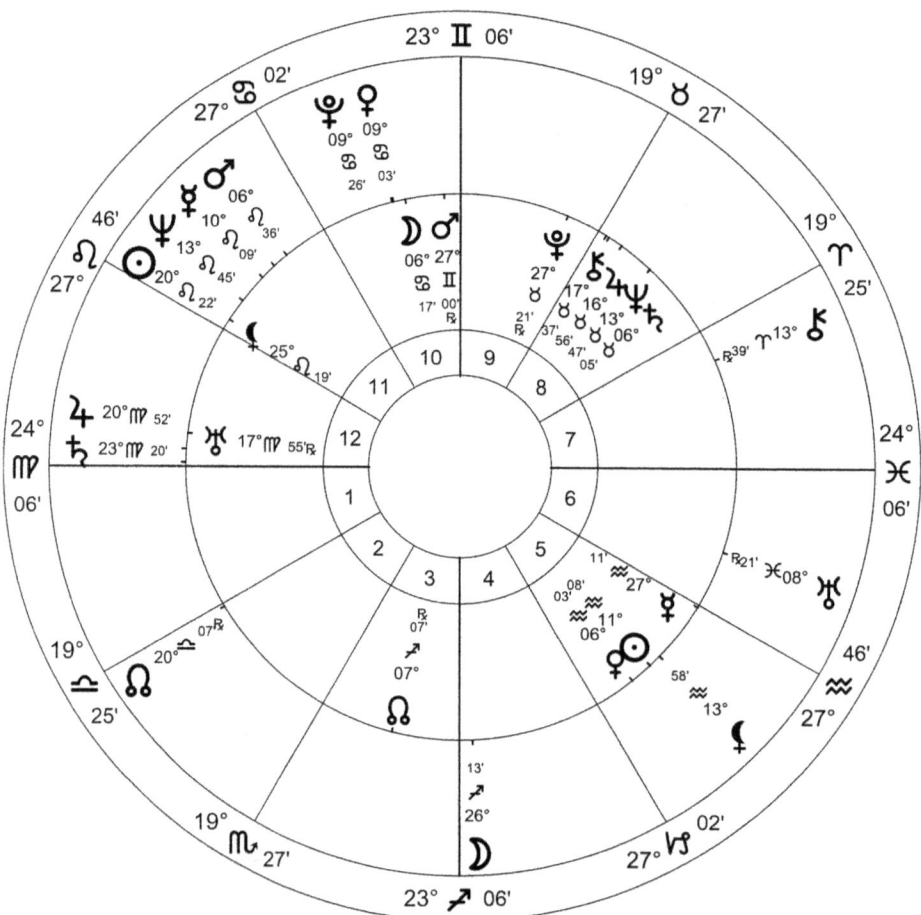

Figure 16. Franklin Roosevelt
Inner Wheel: Natal Chart; Outer Wheel, Transits
Proserpina: ADD DEGREE AND SIGN

I always work with exact aspects only (maximum one-degree orb) as from my experience this is necessary in order to make accurate forecasts. For example, in the case of Franklin Roosevelt I didn't take into consideration a progressed square between Mars and Saturn because it occurred five to six months before the beginning of the disease. This progression certainly could bring problems with the musculoskeletal system, but most likely as a result of injury. In the case of Roosevelt's paralysis, transits and progressions work together perfectly, supporting each other.

Midpoints

I don't use midpoints in my astrological practice. Not because they are of no significance but simply because the techniques I do use work well.

The first time I heard about the use of midpoints in medical astrology was in the early 1990s, at an astrological conference in Moscow. Igor Podolsky, an astrologer and anaesthesiologist with the Krasnodar hospital, made a fascinating presentation about medical astrology. It was especially impressive because Podolsky had collected a vast base of data, and had an opportunity to use astrological knowledge in his clinic to help people

Of course, there was a lot more information in his talk; not just midpoints, though here I'll focus only on them. Igor Podolsky also used planets of the Hamburg school: fictitious planets such as Cupid, Admetos, Zeus and others, which I don't use. However, I think it makes sense to look at midpoints between real planets.

Secondary progressions are used with midpoints, and if a planet reaches a midpoint by secondary progression, this could indicate a certain event (not always an illness).

Below are some midpoints and possible illnesses:

Planet	Midpoint	Possible influence
Saturn	Mars/Pluto	Poisoning by metals
The Sun	Saturn/Pluto	Endocrine system disorders
The Sun	Saturn/Uranus	Nervous exhaustion due to overstrain
Mars	Sun/Moon	Conception
Mars	Mercury/Uranus	Stress
Jupiter	Mars/Neptune	Blood poisoning; hepatitis
Jupiter	Mars/Uranus	Successful surgery
Saturn	Moon/Venus	Barrenness
Neptune	Sun/Jupiter	Medication overdose

The above-mentioned astrologer and physician wrote an astrological dissertation based on statistics he collected through his work. Unfortunately, traditional medical practitioners are too conservative to accept the use of astrology in medicine; we can only hope this will change with time.

Chapter Eleven

The Horoscope of Disease

Just as everything has a distinct beginning, an illness has its own horoscope. The horoscope of disease is called a decumbiture. The question that immediately arises is at which time should the onset of the illness be based. The opinion of astrologers varies widely in this regard, and so we will discuss three kinds of decumbitures.

The first kind of decumbiture is when the illness infiltrates only on the energy level, while on the physical level the person does not yet feel anything.

The second kind of decumbiture is the first sign of symptoms.

The third kind of decumbiture is for the time the patient took to his or her bed.

The First Kind of Decumbiture

It is no great mystery that the onset of illness occurs first on the energy level. The person is still physically healthy, but energy healers already see problems in the patient's aura. In many cases, if caught before it transfers to the physical level—and is treated with energy healing—the disease can be avoided. Unfortunately, this does not apply to a karmic illness.

Constructing a decumbiture of the first kind is incredibly difficult. As you may recall from the case with oncology, an illness can lie dormant for years, and the foundation of the illness usually occurs in the years of evil planets. The years of the Antihyleg are particularly marked. It is believed that the first kind of decumbiture begins with the formation of the exact aspect from a transiting planet to a corresponding planet of the radix in the year of the evil planet. The planet in aspect must be related to the illness; for example, Pluto for cancer. T-squares and grand crosses are especially significant. If the Antihyleg, or an evil planet that rules the year, or both, are involved in these, then the beginning of illness is very likely.

Karmic illnesses often begin during solar or lunar eclipses. Another sign that the illness is of a karmic nature may be the conjunction of a planet (or planets) with the lunar nodes, Lilith, or fixed stars. These illnesses are very difficult to treat. Here, spiritual practices are the best.

Because of the obvious limitations of this method I never construct the first kind of decumbiture. However, I often look at what laid the foundation for the illness, as this is important for subsequent treatment.

The Second Kind of Decumbiture

The basis of the second kind of decumbiture is the initial symptoms: the first signal of the manifestation of the illness. Here again, serious difficulties can arise. After all, who will pay attention to the time of when the first cough occurs, or heaviness in the heart region is felt? It's unlikely, isn't it? However, in some cases this is possible, such as in the case of heavy bleeding.

Let's suppose that we were able to determine the Ascendant and construct a chart. What could this give us? The second kind of decumbiture will help us to see how the illness will progress, as well as suggest which method of treatment to choose.

It is believed that for women it is worse when an illness manifests itself during the day, the yang half of the twenty-four hour period; for men, it is during the night, the ying half of the day. It is also considered a negative indicator if the sign of the sixth house of the personal chart ascends in the horoscope of the illness; this signifies a prolonged illness that is difficult to treat and that takes a lot of strength away from the person. It is good if the sign of the Ascendant ascends; then the illness will pass easily and good health will quickly return.

The ascending sign of the decumbiture roughly indicates the course of the illness. If a fire sign ascends, the course of the illness will be in the acute form; if an earth sign ascends, then the illness will be of a prolonged nature. The Ascendant in an air sign indicates changeable and unclear symptoms with exacerbations and quick improvements. Water signs bring hidden illnesses, prolonged and with possible complications. If any planet ascends in the decumbiture, it must definitely be taken into account as it will be more important than the sign itself.

The phase of the Moon is also significant, and the illness is most difficult to treat if it begins in the phase of the Moon opposite the phase in the natal chart. For example, if the person is born with the Moon in the first quarter, it is unfavourable if he or she becomes ill during the third quarter of the Moon. The opposite of the second quarter is the fourth quarter and so on. It is good if the Moon is in the same phase in the horoscope of disease and the natal chart. The method of treatment with herbs or homeopathy is also determined by the lunar phase: either "similar by similar," or "similar by opposite." We will discuss the subtleties of treatment in more detail in chapter fourteen.

The Third Kind of Decumbiture

The chart is constructed for the moment the person "takes to his bed." Again, it is difficult to determine the exact time, but at least we can learn at what time of day the illness so overwhelmed the patient that he or she was unable to lead a normal lifestyle. The phase of the twenty-four hour period is also tied to the elements and reflects the course of illness.

If the illness rendered the person bedridden in the morning, in the period from sunrise to noon, then likely it will pass by in an acute form, with a high temperature, but will be brief. If it occurred from noon to sunset, the illness is also relatively easy to treat and tends to pass quickly. From sunset to midnight the illness is changeable with periods of exacerbation and improvement; however, this illness could also be relatively prolonged, but not as much as an illness that is manifested from midnight to sunrise. The later illness is severe and lingering.

I almost never calculate decumbitures in my practice because they take a lot of time and achieving accuracy is extremely difficult. However, in the case of severe illness and prolonged treatment, I do turn to the horoscope of disease in order to choose the most effective method of treatment. And as for the prognosis of the course of illness, there is an easier method that is based on lunar days. We will consider it in the next chapter.

Chapter Twelve

Lunar Days

Cycles of the Moon were widely used in ancient times to determine the time for planting in order to get an excellent harvest, for conceiving a child, for preparation of medicine, and for healing. In addition to the phases of the Moon, the lunar days were considered. A new lunar calendar begins at each month's New Moon.

The lunar calendar includes thirty lunar days. Lunar days are not equal in magnitude and they can differ significantly from each other. The lunar month does not coincide with the solar month, with the lunar month being approximately 29.5 sun days. The length of the first lunar day is from the New Moon until the moon rising; therefore, the first lunar day might be very short, sometimes lasting for only a few minutes if, for example, the New Moon occurs just prior to the moon rising. If it is long, then often the lunar month has twenty-nine, not thirty days.

Thus, each lunar day lasts from the rise of the moon until its next rise (except for the New Moon). They are fairly easy to calculate for the place where you live. Do not forget time zones and Daylight Saving Time. Astrological computer programs that calculate lunar days are also available.

Each lunar day has its own symbol and information. The lunar calendar is also used in esoteric astrology for spiritual work. Included here is information on lunar days as they relate to medical astrology and are applied to decumbitures. If you have recorded at least an approximate time of appearance of first symptoms (chest pain, toothache, etc.) of an illness, then the lunar day of the beginning of the illness can give information about the character, course, and possible treatment of the disease.

Below is information about each of the thirty lunar days as it pertains to medical astrology.

First Lunar Day

This is typically a short day. However, if the previous lunar month had only twenty-nine days, a disease of this day can be very treacherous. It is especially bad if the first lunar day occurred after an eclipse because the disease may have a karmic character, thereby requiring treatment by spiritual methods. If the previous lunar month had thirty days (without an eclipse), then the disease will be facile and does not need to be treated; it will heal by itself.

Second Lunar Day

The course of a disease depends upon how many days there were in the previous lunar month. If twenty-nine, the disease can take away a lot of strength and develop in the most unexpected places. Eating a lot is not recommended if you become ill in the second lunar day. The less food, the better; the more food absorbed, the worse your physical condition could become. Even poisoning can happen. A strict diet and herbal therapy are best for this day. It also makes sense to recall what you ate before you became ill and to eliminate those products from the menu because they could be illness-provokers. This is especially important for people with allergies and those who suffer from stomach and liver diseases.

Third Lunar Day

Diseases of this day usually have an acute character, but they pass quickly. They have clear symptoms and heal easily. Women who contract an illness in the third lunar day typically feel much worse than men.

This day is associated with metals, including iron, and is considered to be auspicious for surgery (if there are no contraindications).

Fourth Lunar Day

This day is associated with karma, including hereditary karma. Thus, diseases of this day can be karmic or genetic, namely those that are not easily treated (especially by traditional means). Diseases of the fourth day can be very long lasting. They are rarely acute; however, they have one unpleasant trait: they tend to transfer into a chronic phase. A person can get used to such a disease to the point where it will become a part of everyday life.

Diseases of this day are not recommended for treatment only with traditional methods (though they are not contraindicated). Prayers are very helpful here. Water and liquids in general also play a big role in the recovery process.

Fifth Lunar Day

Diseases of this day are a proof of toxins in the body, and those who become ill on this day have accumulated a lot of toxins. It is the right time to start ridding the body of them. Everything is important here: clean air, proper diet, positive thinking. The more strictly you follow these rules the faster you will recover.

Ailments of the fifth day progress more in older people than in young ones. Children generally do not get sick on this day because their level of toxins is much lower.

Sixth Lunar Day

Diseases of the sixth lunar day are difficult to treat because they have complex and intricate symptoms. There is a clear danger of misdiagnosis and it is not unusual for the person to be treated for the wrong thing. It is reasonable to carefully double-check the diagnosis, especially where surgery is concerned. Sometimes while undergoing surgery the reason for the procedure cannot be found.

Women are subject to diseases of this day more easily than men. These illnesses should be taken seriously: if they are not fully healed, they easily become chronic.

Seventh Lunar Day

Diseases of the seventh day can also be treacherous. Do not engage in self-treatment: an experienced physician is needed. These diseases usually have an acute form, which in this case is good because the result will be that they pass faster. If the disease is prolonged it can become chronic, so it is wise to proceed with active treatment from the beginning. If antibiotics are needed, a loading dose should be taken at the beginning for a short term. It is important to have positive thinking on the seventh lunar day. If you talk and think less about the disease, you will recover much faster.

Eighth Lunar Day

Diseases of the eighth day can be quite difficult. However, the more acute the beginning of the disease, the faster a person improves. If you have a high temperature, do not panic: diseases with a fever will pass faster. If your heart allows, the temperature should not be lowered. If you do not have a fever but the condition is painful, recovery might take longer than planned. Cleansing of the whole body can be beneficial on this lunar day.

Ninth Lunar Day

The ninth lunar day is one of the toughest and called a "Satanic" day by the Avestan Astrological School. Diseases of this day might have a strange, mystical nature. Random diseases cannot happen on the ninth lunar day. These illnesses are proof of contamination, including a karmic one. They can also be a manifestation of a hereditary curse.

These diseases can almost never be cured by traditional methods and a serious approach is required. Recovery is in the hands of the patient and his or her relatives. Blood-related people can be really helpful, even by just being there. Lonesome people have a harder time; family people always take illnesses easier. Care and concern for the loved one are necessary here.

Additionally, dairy products are helpful with diseases of this day. Fever is a bad sign. The body responds well to application of ice (but only in small amounts).

Tenth Lunar Day

Diseases of this day are associated with hereditary karma and are strongly tied to the subconscious mind: fears and childhood complexes that have been driven into the depths of the subconscious can appear on the physical level. Diseases of the tenth day more severely affect people who do not have a regular sex life; married or committed people recover faster. Also, diseases of this day might be the result of poor life choices and represent a push for changing the lifestyle to a healthier one.

Heat or cold do not matter for the tenth day. However, water is very important. It is very useful to drink spring or mineral water. Sauna is also beneficial.

Eleventh Lunar Day

Diseases of this day are strong, affecting the entire body and consuming a lot of energy. However, if they begin abruptly, they leave quickly. Unfortunately, ailments of the eleventh day often become repetitive. For example, renal colic that occurred on this day can quickly disappear and the person will forget about it; but it could return after a few months.

Diseases of the eleventh day have a negative effect on blood formulation, especially on hemoglobin. This is why it is necessary to check the blood periodically and, if needed, take medication to improve the level of hemoglobin. Antibiotics should not be over-prescribed, especially for people suffering from anaemia.

Twelfth Lunar Day

If you became ill on the twelfth lunar day, consider yourself lucky: the disease passes easily and quickly and is not repetitive. It is best to get a lot of rest: stay in bed without moving. Alcohol might be useful on this day (in reasonable quantities, of course).

Thirteenth Lunar Day

Diseases of this day are severe, lingering, recurring, and difficult to treat. Try to remember the circumstances under which you became ill: what did you eat and drink, with whom did you communicate, and the active stressors in your life. If the illness returns there is a big chance it will return under the same circumstances. If you can eliminate these circumstances from your life, then you will not become ill.

Fourteenth Lunar Day

Diseases of this day are just the beginning of a chain of other ailments that could be very different. For example, the illness could begin with a cough, followed by stomach ache, then cardiac arrhythmia, etc. Illnesses of the fourteenth day require complex treatment. This is a case where you need to treat not the illness (meaning symptoms) but the patient. Take a serious approach to the treatment protocol.

Fifteenth Lunar Day

This is a difficult one: another of the so-called "Satanic" days. Diseases of this day are often associated with the evil-eye and curses, which are always related to negative energy. There are many reasons for someone to wish evil upon you: jealousy is first on the list, along with anger, debt, workplace difficulties, etc. As a result, the first symptom is loss of energy, after which you might become ill.

These diseases cannot be cured by ordinary methods. Here we need special procedures such as cleansing rituals. With their help, negative energy is removed from the aura. Healing is much easier if the previous lunar month had thirty days. If there were twenty-nine days, it is much more complicated. Praying, fasting, and avoiding negative thoughts are useful here.

Since the fifteenth lunar day falls on a Full Moon, it is overall a good time for body cleansings, including a mental one through meditation and prayers.

Sixteenth Lunar Day

On this day the most attention should be directed to the mental state because diseases of the sixteenth day usually are psychosomatic. Symptoms on the physical level merely reflect the emotional state. For example, you have stomachache even though there are no changes on the physical level; it is just your sadness, depression, or nervous agitation showing. Or, for example, people who are angry and irritable often suffer from gallbladder disorders. If you treat only the symptoms, but not the mental state, the disease will not disappear. Help from a therapist might be good. Self-hypnosis and meditation also work very well here.

Seventeenth Lunar Day

Diseases of this day are acute and have a prolonged course with simple and clear symptoms. The more relaxed you are on this day, the faster you will improve. On the seventeenth lunar day, drinking wine, especially red wine, is considered very helpful. On this day wine brings maximum benefit (when consumed in reasonable quantities).

Eighteenth Lunar Day

Diseases of this day are insidious with unstable and misleading symptoms. The possibility of a medical error is likely, resulting in treatment for the wrong disease. Be very careful with medication as there is a high risk of side effects. Drug allergy for women usually affects the respiratory system. For men it will mostly have an effect on skin. Even poisoning from a drug overdose is possible.

Nineteenth Lunar Day

Diseases of this day are serious. Treatment should not be delayed; medicine should be taken immediately. It is better not to do any surgery (even urgent) on this day because there could be serious complications. Illnesses of the nineteenth day are insidious. Even if you think the disease is cured, it can return in another form. Energy healing works well for diseases of this day.

Twentieth Lunar Day

Illnesses of this day largely depend on environment. An unpleasant psychological climate in the family or at work could trigger ailments. Older people deal with them a lot more easily than do younger ones. The ailment can be lingering and requires patience; the disease will reach its peak and slowly subside. The treatment regimen should be strictly obeyed. Multiple treatment methods should not be tried at the same time; choose one and do not change it. Also, do not change your physician.

Twenty-first Lunar Day

Diseases of this day are simple with clear symptoms. If you become ill while traveling, the sickness will progress more easily than if you become ill at home. You should not spend much time in bed on the twenty-first lunar day. It is better to be active as in this way a faster recovery can be expected. These diseases are not repetitive.

Twenty-second Lunar Day

Illnesses of this day can be very difficult, long-lasting, and strength-consuming, ultimately evolving into the chronic phase. It is necessary to find a competent physician in addition to self-treatment. In this case it is even useful to read a medical encyclopaedia: the more you know about the disease the more efficiently you can help yourself.

Twenty-third Lunar Day

This is one of the most negative days, sometimes called a "crocodile day." It is a poor day to become ill, and especially to be injured, and is unfavorable for surgery. You should not depend only on physicians on this day as there is a high probability of a medical error. In general, the less you communicate with people on the twenty-third day, the better.

Twenty-fourth Lunar Day

Diseases of this day are exhausting and lingering. They may worsen the overall condition of the body and affect blood formulation. It is best to prepare from the beginning for a long and persistent treatment.

Weight loss is considered a bad sign; therefore, it is especially important to eat nutritious foods. It is good to sleep a lot in order to gain strength, and to take fewer drugs, instead focusing more on natural products that enhance resistance.

Twenty-fifth Lunar Day

If on this day the disease affects an organ or body part, it will be localized and will not transfer to other organs. The disease has simple symptoms but needs laborious treatment. Illnesses of the twenty-fifth day can be treated well by traditional medicine. Following a physician's guidance can enhance recovery.

The woman whose chart is shown in Figure 10 (chapter ten), became ill on the twenty-fifth lunar day. Despite being a serious oncological disease, it was successfully treated, and the tumor has not metastasized. The treatment was based on the system existing at that time: surgery followed by radiation therapy. The recovery was complete (excluding some side effects of radiation).

Twenty-sixth Lunar Day

Diseases of this day often produce false symptoms and as a result of improper treatment they could transfer into a chronic form. A comprehensive treatment of the whole body and not just of the symptoms is required.

Latent forms of cancer can occur on the twenty-sixth lunar day. Surgery performed on this day could lead to the degeneration of tissues (same as on the nineteenth lunar day); therefore, treatment needs to be done cautiously.

Twenty-seventh Lunar Day

Ailments of this day are simple. Symptoms may be vague but amenable to psychotherapy and energy healing. It is good to drink plenty of fluids, and sauna and massage work well here. Generally, older people recover faster than younger people.

The blood formula should be checked so as not to miss any changes. X-rays are not recommended on this day because the irradiation can have an immediate side effect not only on blood but also on potency for men.

Twenty-eighth Lunar Day

Diseases of this day are serious and often have a karmic nature. Doctors are not much help here: your recovery is in your hands. Use multiple techniques in your effort to understand the cause of the illness; generally it lies very deep inside. You could use meditation on chakras and meditation for recovery and raising the body's defenses. Treatment should be carried out using your intuition, asking your body (and your soul) what it needs. Be prepared for it to take a lot of time and discipline.

Twenty-ninth Lunar Day

This is one of the most difficult so-called "Satanic" days. People who become ill on this day have a weak astral protection or are easily influenced. These people easily absorb the negative energy impact that comes from the environment. The key to successful treatment is privacy: no visitors, and communicate only with your physician.

Cleansing of the entire body using a variety of methods is helpful. Procedures that cleanse the aura might involve energy healing, water, wax, or clay. Prayers and meditation are helpful. It is better to avoid surgery on this day because it could lead to unexpected and adverse results. Only an absolutely spiritually pure doctor should perform surgery on this day.

Thirtieth Lunar Day

The thirtieth lunar day does not happen every month and often does not last long. Diseases of this day are not simple, and they are a reminder of our spiritual deficiencies, with their roots in the distant past. They are treated only with spiritual methods. Medication is useless. Water treatments are good, as is cleansing the body.

The diseases of the thirtieth day are not lingering in nature and if you manage to get rid of one, it will not return. The last day of the lunar month is excellent for rejuvenation.

Chapter Thirteen

The Moon in the Signs

Choosing the Proper Time for Surgery and Much More

In many countries patients do not have a choice of date and time for surgery, even if it is not urgent. (The information here does not pertain to emergency procedures.) Even in the case of a planned surgery, when a physician appoints the date, it's hard to disagree with it. If one has to wait several months for the surgery, one is happy just to have the date set.

However, in half of the cases, where a few possible days are offered, we do have a choice, and it is sometimes better to wait a little longer in order to choose the right date and time. Ancient physicians always took notice of the lunar rhythm, and although they lacked much of what modern medicine has to offer, among them were some eminent individuals. Choosing the correct date and time can decrease the probability of medical error and unwanted consequences, and also accelerate the recovery period. Dr. Podolsky (see chapter ten) collected amazing statistics on this topic.

In order to seriously approach the subject, a professional astrologer would need to look at the horoscope of the patient. But even without this, simply knowing the natural cycles is very helpful.

Each part of the human body corresponds to a particular sign of the zodiac. Figure 1 (chapter one) clearly depicts this correlation.

The head, except for the lower jaw, is ruled by Aries. The lower jaw and the neck, as well as all the internal organs (trachea, tonsils, etc.) are ruled by Taurus. Shoulders, collarbone, arms, and bronchi belong to Gemini. Cancer rules the chest and the mammary glands. For Leo, it is the spine. The abdominal cavity belongs to Virgo. The small of the back and the kidneys are ruled by Libra. Scorpio rules the reproductive organs and the anus. Sagittarius rules the buttocks and hips. For Capricorn, it is the knees; for Aquarius, the shins. Pisces rules the feet.

There is a general rule: one should not have surgey on the part of the body ruled by the sign in which the Moon is located *at the moment of surgery*. Although one shouldn't have surgery on the part of the body or organ of the sign in which the Moon is located, the parts of the body of the opposite sign are in a strong position and may undergo procedures.

Moon in Aries

During the transit of the Moon through Aries, it is not recommended to perform surgery on the head or face (including cosmetic surgery.) Teeth shouldn't be removed. In fact, it is better to postpone seeing a dentist. One shouldn't have the ears pierced or even get a haircut. The head and eyes are vulnerable during this period. Headaches can arise from fatigue and overconcentration, which is why during this period excessive computer time or reading is not recommended.

It is believed that when the Moon is in Aries the organs of the opposite sign, Libra, function well, namely the kidneys and the bladder. Performing surgery, as well as non-surgical procedures (for example, acupuncture) on these organs is not contraindicated.

Moon in Taurus

In this case the throat and endocrine system are vulnerable. Throat and neck surgeries shouldn't be performed (for example, removing tonsils). Additionally, sensitivity to food is heightened and the choice of food should be carefully considered. With the Moon in Taurus, one should not fast.

Surgery on the organs of the opposite sign, Scorpio (genitals), can be done. However, endocrinal glands shouldn't be touched.

Moon in Gemini

Shoulders and arms become vulnerable. Lung and bronchi surgeries are contraindicated at this time. Breathing practices are also not recommended (Pranayama, for example), with one exception: when the Sun is also located in this air sign. Sensitivity to air pollution may also become heightened, and intolerance of stuffy rooms may arise. One should strive to increase exposure to fresh air, and smokers should reduce their consumption of cigarettes.

With the Moon in Gemini, blood and liver cleansing procedures are favorable.

Moon in Cancer

Stomach and mammary gland surgeries are contraindicated. The acidity of gastric juices undergoes changes during this period: it rises for those born during daytime and falls for those with a nighttime birth. It's important to watch your diet carefully, excluding chemical additives and alcohol as much as possible. Energy healing is not recommended.

With the Moon in Cancer it's a good time to remove stones and toxins from the body, including the treatment of arthritis. Treating or removing teeth, and having leg, knee, joint, or tendon surgery is acceptable. Treating metabolic illnesses, including adopting prophylactic measures, is also favorable.

Moon in Leo

As the heart is weakened during this period, it is not a good idea to overburden the heart nor to overstrain oneself in general. Try to spend your energy thoughtfully. Surgeries on the heart and spine should be avoided.

Treating vascular illnesses, the nervous system, and the organs of sight is favorable. One could also have joint or shin surgeries.

Moon in Virgo

The gastrointestinal tract is vulnerable (except for the rectum), which is why during these days it is important to pay attention to maintaining a healthy diet. All surgery on the abdominal cavity is contraindicated.

Blood and liver cleansing procedures are favorable during this period, as well as the treatment of skin diseases. It is also an excellent time for cosmetic procedures and preparation for cosmetic surgery, although it is better to have the surgery performed when the Moon enters the next sign: Libra.

Moon in Libra

The kidneys should not be overstrained during this time. The urinary and endocrine systems, pancreas, and skin are fairly vulnerable. The skin suffers mainly because toxins are poorly excreted from the body. If suffering from diabetes or pancreatitis, one should be more careful with diet during this time. Eating foods that are hard to digest (when the Moon is in Libra) causes the pancreas to make itself known the next day, and illness may be exacerbated.

When the Moon is in Libra, comsetic surgery can be performed on the face as well as on other parts of the head (ears, for example.) Teeth can be removed.

Moon in Scorpio

Reproductive organ surgery is not recommended. For women who are prone to disruptions in their menstrual cycle, these problems can be aggravated with the Moon in Scorpio. The rectum is also related to Scorpio, and therefore hemorrhoid removal surgery is also not recommended at this time. With the Moon in this position, consuming spicy foods is also not recommended, as hemorrhoids may worsen and constipation may result.

The endocrine system can be treated at this time (with the exception of the prostate), as well as sinuses, throat, and upper respiratory tract. Tonsils and adenoid glands can be removed.

Moon in Sagittarius

The liver is not strong during this time, so liver and gallbladder surgery is contraindicated, as are blood transfusions and donor procedures. Surgery on the parts of the body ruled by Sagittarius is also not recommended: hips and hip joints (problems with the sciatic nerve are also included).

Lung treatment is permitted, as are all the related supporting procedures. Breathing practices are beneficial.

Moon in Capricorn

All surgery connected to the teeth, spine, and joints is contraindicated (all joints, not just knees). It can be dangerous to see manual therapists (chiropractors) while the Moon is in Capricorn, as unwanted side effects and even medical errors can arise.

Procedures related to the stomach and the diaphragm are recommended. In principle, with this position of the Moon one can eat anything without denying oneself any kind of tasty food.

Moon in Aquarius

With the transit of the Moon through Aquarius, shin surgery (for example, removal of varicose veins) is contraindicated. Also, with the night luminary in this position, the nervous system and the sensory organs (especially eyesight) are vulnerable and thus should not be disturbed.

Procedures related to the element of air (breathing practices, for example) are not recommended; however, all water procedures are very favourable. Nevertheless, if you are planning cold water therapy in order to strengthen the immune system, it might be a good idea to first see if there are important planets (the Sun, for example) in the sixth house of the horoscope. If they are there, then this prophylactic therapy should be approached with much caution.

With the Moon in Aquarius, physical exercise is recommended; it's good to make the heart and the cardiovascular system work and increase blood circulation.

Moon in Pisces

With the Moon in this position it is not recommended to consume a lot of liquids (including alcohol) as there is a tendency for tissue to retain liquids. Surgery on the feet is contraindicated. With the Moon in Pisces, the risk of allergies increases (including drug allergies), and so do problems with the skin and blood.

One also shouldn't walk excessively as the feet are more sensitive than usual. In any case, comfortable footwear is needed. One should also refrain from foot massage. Water procedures are not recommended, and care should be taken with medication.

During these days, with the help of a proper diet, a variety of illnesses can be successfully treated.

Please remember, nothing is simple in medical astrology as it relates directly to our health and life in general. *It is not enough to know only the Moon position in signs for successful surgery.* If you want to use astrological knowledge in the medical area, it is necessary to see a professional astrologer who specializes in this branch of astrology. You personal chart should be taken into consideration as well as the transits of many planets, including Mars, Saturn, Uranus, and Neptune. Neptune should be always considered because its position is responsible for any complications with anesthesia.

Chapter Fourteen

Using Medical Astrology in Healing Practice

This chapter focuses on the use of astrological knowledge in the treatment of illness, not just in diagnosis. We will consider naturopathy (herbs), energy healing, and achieving a lifestyle to the prevent ailments.

The application of healing plants requires comprehensive knowledge. *Note that after reading this chapter you will not be able to confidently use this method.* For this it is necessary to take a special course of naturopathy or to extensively study books about herbs. The addition of astrology to herbal healing gives knowledge that multiplies the effectiveness of this kind of treatment.

Every plant contains a specific energy that is related to planetary influences—sometimes one planet, more often two or three. As you recall from previous chapters, planets are associated with illnesses, life systems, and organs. We can thus use plants to strengthen or heal organs. However, it isn't as simple as it might seem.

First, we need to choose between two treatment methods: "similar by similar" and "similar by opposite." The first method is based on the use of herbs of the same planet as the ruler of the ailing organ (herbs will make the organ stronger). For example, burdock or cranberry for improving the liver's condition (they all are ruled by Jupiter). The method "similar by opposite" is based on damping down the strength of the planet responsible for the illness. In this case plants of the planet-antagonist are applied. For example, for headaches and haemorrhoids, herbs of Venus can be used in order to weaken Mars' power, which is responsible for these illnesses.

Below is a list of planets-antagonists.

- Sun-Moon
- Venus-Mars

- Jupiter-Saturn
- Mercury-Jupiter
- Uranus-Jupiter
- Neptune-Mars
- Proserpina-Jupiter
- Pluto-Venus

Which of the two methods should be chosen is a rather difficult question. It is necessary to pay attention to decumbiture and the progression of the disease. If the illness develops slowly, it makes sense to choose "similar by similar" to strengthen the impaired organ. If the illness is in an acute phase, use "similar by opposite" to alleviate the patient's suffering.

There is another rule that is based on the position of planets regarding the Sun. In this regard planets subdivide into eastern and western. Eastern planets are located before the Sun, i.e. they ascend before the Sun; western planets ascend after the Sun. If the planet ruling the ill organ is eastern, then the method "similar by similar" is more appropriate. If it is western, use "similar by opposite." However, if there are any doubts as to which of the approaches should be chosen, always give preference to "similar by similar."

Second, identify the correct time to pick herbs as well as to make and take medicine. (This topic is discussed later.) Now we need to clarify the division of plants into groups according to their containing energy of specific planets.

Plant Types

Plants of the Sun are notable for their bright flowers, mostly yellow or golden color, round forms, and hard stalks and leaves. The Sun's trees are tall and straight with a luxuriant crown. These plants have no, or very weak, fragrance. Calendula is the only exception, but this is because it has a touch of Venus. In addition to calendula the typical herbs of the Sun are buttercup, coltsfoot, dandelion, bur-marigold, celandine, St. John's Wort, and chamomile. The magic plants of the Sun are the sunflower and the poplar tree.

Plants that contain a lot of liquid are ruled by the Moon and include the many marsh and lake herbs (water lilies). The Moon's plants have fleshy stalks and leaves with flowers that are mostly white. Edible plants are melon, watermelon, cucumber, pumpkin, and coconut. The Moon's trees like to grow near water, and the typical Moon tree is willow. Magic plants of the Moon are white water lily and lotus.

Plants of Mercury are creeping herbs (bindweed, pea, hop, knot-grass). All of them have small, thin stalks and small variegated flowers. The magic plant of Mercury is mistletoe (from the birch tree).

Venus herbs have a strong and pleasant scent. Their flowers are lilac or violet, sometimes white:

violet, sage, origanum, chamerion (rose-bay), lilac, jasmine, lily-of-the-valley (with the addition of the Moon's energy), bird cherry tree, and the linden tree (with addition of the Sun). Venus rules many fruit trees with sweet fruits: apple, peach, and pear, for example. Venus herbs are also used in cosmetology. Magic plants of Venus are jasmine and orchids.

Mars plants have a tough temperament: thorny, sharp, or burning (sedge, thistle, nettle, saggitaria). Hot plants and hot spicy relishes also belong to Mars (pepper, onion, garlic). There are many poisonous herbs as well, such as henbane. Mars is present in all plants that have thorns. Roses, for example, contain energies of Mars and Venus. Cacti take their fleshy stalk from the Moon and their thorns from Mars. The magic Mars plant is nettle.

Plants of Jupiter are large. Trees are tall and strong-looking (oak, baobab). Herbs of Jupiter have a thick, hollow stalk (burdock, angelica, rhubarb), or are umbellate herbs (yarrow, tansy, dill, cilantro, caraway). The taste of Jupiter's fruits and berries is sour (cranberry, cowberry). Magic plants of Jupiter are oak and yarrow.

Saturn herbs are dry with a bitter taste (wormwood, immortelle, field horsetail). The stalks are always straight, not creeping. All relic plants are ruled by Saturn: horsetail, ferns, heather, and all evergreen conifers (fir; thuja; cypress; pine, with the Sun). Plants of Saturn usually have dark seeds with an astringent taste. The magic plants are cypress and heather.

Among Uranus plants we can find herbs being carried by the wind (like tumbleweed) as well as some plant parasites (with the exception of mushrooms). There are also some plants that look like Mercury plants: lianas and schisandra (magnolia vine). Uranus rules moss and lichen.

All algae, including seaweed (such as laminaria) and weeds from lakes and rivers (duckweed), are ruled by Neptune.

Mushrooms belong to Pluto. Chaga mushroom is a medicinal mushroom famous because it is a powerful medicine for preventing and treating cancer (in the early stage).

Plants of Proserpina are plant mutants or hybrids (for example, grapefruit).

Chiron has not been studied and therefore isn't used.

The above is a general classification. Few plants contain the power of only one planet, instead combining the influences and power of several planets. You can read more about this below.

Planetary Energy in Plants and Time for Collecting Herbs

It is much easier to purchse herbs, but there is no guarantee as to their quality or if they were properly gatheed. Herb picking is an art. In addition to the right time there are a few other rules with regard to harvesting herbs for medical treatment. I won't mention all of them but will mention a few important ones. It is best not to use metal tools in picking herbs; wooden or ivory tools are better or use your hands. Your thoughts should be pure and you need to talk to the plants, apologize for picking them, and ask for their healing help.

There is a whole system with regard to timing when it comes to harvesting herbs, but some general rules about the correct time to pick herbs are included here. Leaves, flowers, and stems should be picked on the waxing Moon, and roots should be dug out on the waning moon. Herbs of the Sun, Moon, Mercury, and Venus should be collected on the waxing Moon, while plants of Mars, Saturn, Jupiter, and Neptune should be picked on the waning Moon. Harvesting of Uranus and Pluto plants can be in any Moon phase, just not at the time of the exact aspects, meaning that luminaries shouldn't be in exact conjunction, square, or opposition.

Below is a list of different plants with their rules and the right time for picking. Though not every plant will be found in your area, some of them will definitely be there.

Acorus: Contains power of Saturn, Jupiter, Mars, and the Moon. Acorus leaves are gathered in the First Quarter lunar phase around sunrise. The roots are dug out in the Third Quarter close to sunset.

Angelica: This is a complicated herb, containing the power of Uranus, Jupiter, Moon, and Sun. It should be picked in the Second Quarter closer to the Full Moon, better on the thirteenth or fourteenth lunar days, after sunset. The timing will be ideal if in addition the Moon is in Gemini or Taurus.

Anis (pimpinella anisum): Contains the power of Uranus and Mercury. It is collected in the First Quarter lunar phase at noon.

Apple Tree: Energies of Venus, Moon, and Jupiter. Apples are gathered on the waxing Moon around noon.

Arnica: Ruled by the Sun and Jupiter. Pick in the First Quarter around sunrise.

Ash-tree: Contains the power of the Sun and Saturn. Flowers and buds are collected in the Fourth Quarter close to the New Moon, before sunset.

Aspen: Contains the Sun, Jupiter, and Mars. Buds, leaves, and branches are collected in the Third Quarter after sunset.

Barberry: Venus, Mars, and Saturn. Berries are harvested in the Third Quarter right after sunset.

Bay-tree: Contains the power of the Sun and Saturn. Pick on the thirteenth and fourteenth lunar days at noon (better when the Sun is in Pisces and the Moon is in Aquarius).

Beans: Contains the power of Venus and Mercury. Harvest on the waxing Moon after sunrise.

Bearberry (arctostaphylos): Energies of Mercury, Venus, and Mars. Pick on the first half of a day in the Full Moon.

Beet: Contains the power of Jupiter, Saturn, Sun, and Moon. Gather in the Third Quarter close to sunset.

Bergenia: Energy of Jupiter and Saturn. Bergenia's roots are dug out around midnight on the waning Moon.

Bilberry: Contains the power of Venus, Saturn, Mercury, and Jupiter. Berries are picked before the New Moon in the morning, leaves in the Third Quarter before sunrise.

Birch Tree: Ruled by the Sun and Moon. Birch leaves are collected in the First Quarter in the morning after sunrise. Birch gets its biggest power close to summer solstice, so if the First Quarter Moon coincides with June 20-22, there isn't a better time to pick. Birch juice is collected on the thirteenth and fourteenth lunar days. The most healing juice can be received when the Sun moves from Aries to Taurus (end of April). Birch buds are picked on the waxing Moon in the morning.

Bird Cherry (Hackberry): This is a complicated tree: Venus, Moon, Mercury, Jupiter, and Saturn. Berries are collected on the waxing Moon close to sunset.

Black Elderberry: Contains Uranus, Mars, Saturn, and the Moon. Flowers, leaves, and berries are picked on the waxing Moon from sunrise until noon. Careful: some parts can be poisonous!

Blackberry: Contains energies of Saturn, Mercury, Mars, and a little bit of Jupiter. Pick in the Third Quarter from noon till sunset.

Blueberry: Saturn, Mercury, Jupiter, and Uranus. Berries are picked in the Second Quarter around the Full Moon, close to sunset.

Buckthorn: Contains the power of Mercury, Saturn, and Mars. Branches and bark are collected in the Third Quarter at sunset, in shade.

Burdock: This is a plant of Jupiter. Leaves are picked in the First Quarter from sunrise until noon. Roots are dug out starting from the middle of September in the waning Moon at sunset.

Cabbage: Contains the energy of the Moon and Jupiter. Gather on the waxing Moon before noon.

Calendula: This is the typical herb of the Sun. Flowers should be picked in the First Quarter right after the New Moon, at noon, in clear, sunny weather. Roots are dug out in the Third Quarter lunar phase at sunset.

Chamomile: Contains the Sun, Moon, and Mercury. Pick in the First Quarter at the morning dew, in sunny weather.

Capsella: Mercury, Jupiter, and a bit of the Sun. Pick in the First Quarter from sunrise until noon.

Carduus: A plant of Mars and Saturn. Pick on the waning Moon after sunset.

Carrot: Contains power of Mars, Saturn, and the Sun. Dig out on the waning Moon, around sunset.

Carum: Contains Uranus, Venus, and Mercury. Pick on the waxing Moon at sunset.

Celandine: This is a complicated herb: the Sun, Mars, Moon, and Proserpina. Pick in the Third Quarter close to sunset. It is better to collect plants that grow in shade.

Centaurea: Saturn, Venus, and a little bit of Jupiter. Pick in the First Quarter right after sunrise.

Chaga Mushroom: This mushroom grows on trees. Contains the power of Pluto with the addition of Mercury. Pick before sunrise close to the Full Moon (thirteenth to fourteenth lunar days). This is the only healing plant of Pluto and of course it is used to cure cancer.

Cherry: Contains the energy of Jupiter and Venus. Pick in the First Quarter from sunrise unil noon.

Chestnut: This is the tree of Jupiter and Venus. Pick in the Second and Third Quarters close to the Full Moon from sunrise until noon.

Chicory: Venus, Jupiter, and a bit of Saturn. Herb should be picked in the Second Quarter close to the Full Moon at noon. Roots are dug out before sunrise on the waning Moon.

Cilantro: Uranus, Mercury, and Venus. Herb and seeds should be picked in the First Quarter around noon.

Coltsfoot (Tussilaga Farfara): Contains the Sun and a bit of Mercury. Pick at sunrise in the First Quarter.

Comfrey (Symphytum Officinale): Contains Venus, Jupiter, and Saturn. Collect before sunrise on the waxing Moon.

Common Knotgrass (birdweed): This is Mercury's plant. Pick in the Second Quarter before sunrise.

Corn: Contains the Sun, Jupiter, and Uranus. Harvest in the Second Quarter close to the Full Moon at sunset.

Cranberry: Contains the energy of Jupiter, Mars, and a little bit of Mercury. Harvest on the waxing Moon during two hours after sunrise or two hours before sunset.

Cucumber: The Moon with the addition of the Sun. Pick on the waxing Moon before sunrise.

Currant: All kinds of currant (red, black, and white) contain the energies of Mercury, Jupiter, and Mars. Black currant also has Saturn and white currant the Moon. Pick at noon on the twelfth, thirteenth, and fourteenth lunar days.

Cypress: This is a pure Saturn energy. Pick in the Second Quarter close to the Full Moon from sunrise until noon. Cypress energy becomes the strongest when the Sun is in Pisces and the Moon in Cancer.

Dandelion: Contains the energy of the Sun and a little bit of Proserpina. Flowers and leaves are picked on the waxing Moon close to sunrise. Roots are dug out in the Third Quarter at sunset; better when the Sun is in the last decan of Virgo.

Dill: Uranus, Mercury, and Venus. Pick in the first half of the day on the waxing Moon.

Drosera (Sundews): One of the rare plants of Proserpina with addition of Uranus and Venus. Pick before sunrise close to the Full Moon.

Fennel: Uranus, Venus, and the Sun. Seeds are collected in the third quarter from sunrise till noon.

Fir: Contains Saturn, Mars, and Jupiter. Needles are picked on the waxing Moon in the morning; corns on the thirteenth and fourteenth moon days after sunset.

Fireweed (Great Willow-herb): This is a Venus herb. Pick on the waxing Moon from sunrise until noon; the best time is when the Moon is in Leo.

Fragaria (Wild Strawberry): Venus, Mercury, Jupiter, and a bit of the Sun. Leaves are collected in the second lunar phase before noon. Berries are picked in the morning dew on the waxing Moon.

Galangal (Alpinia Officinalis): Contains Mercury, Saturn, and the Sun. Galangal's roots are dug out in the fourth quarter close to the New Moon at sunset.

Garlic: Contains the power of Mars with the addition of the Moon and Saturn. Garlic shoots are picked on the waxing Moon from sunrise until noon. Cloves are dug out on the sixteenth and seventeenth moon days close to sunset. Garlic is a very strong medicine for many illnesses.

Gooseberry: Contains energy of Mars, Venus, and Jupiter. Pick in the Third Quarter, on the sixteenth and seventeenth moon days at the morning dew.

Grapes: Contains the Sun and Mars. Harvest in the first lunar phase from sunrise until noon.

Heather: This is a pure Saturn plant. Collect in the Fourth Quarter, close to the New Moon.

Hazelnut and Walnut: Energies of Jupiter, the Sun, and Saturn. Pick right after the New Moon at sunset.

Hornbeam: The Sun and Jupiter. Collect on the waxing Moon from sunrise until noon.

Horsetail: Contains energies of Uranus and Mercury. Pick on the waning Moon at sunset.

Horseradish: Contains power of Saturn, Jupiter, and Mars. Roots can be dug out any time around sunset. The only limitation is that there should not be a square or opposition between the Sun and the Moon.

Immortelle (helichrysum arenarium): Energies of the Sun and Saturn. Only the upper part of the herb is picked; do this in the first quarter at noon.

Inula: Contains power of the Sun with the addition of Mars and Jupiter energy. Flowers are picked at noon in the first lunar quarter or at sunset in the second lunar phase.

Juniper: Contains energies of Saturn, Mercury, and the Sun. Juniper berries are collected on the waxing Moon around the Full Moon (the thirteenth and fourteenth lunar days) close to sunset.

Lamium (Deadnettle): Contains power of Venus and Mars. Pick in the Third Quarter around sunset.

Larch: Contains powers of Saturn, the Moon, and Jupiter. Collected on the thirteenth and fourteenth lunar days around sunset.

Lavender: This is the herb of Venus. Pick on the waxing Moon at sunrise.

Medical Astrology for Healing

Ledum: Contains powers of Venus and Saturn. Collect in the Third Quarter around the Full Moon (sixteenth and seventeenth lunar days) at noon. The best time for picking is when the Sun is in the last decan of Leo or the first decan of Virgo.

Lemon: Contains energy of Jupiter with the addition of the Sun and Venus. Gathered in the Second Quarter close to the Full Moon from sunrise till noon.

Lilac: This is a plant of Venus. White lilac has an addition of the Moon's energy. Flowers are picked on the waxing Moon at noon.

Liquorice (Gliycyrehize): Contains power of Venus with the addition of Saturn. Roots are dug out in the third lunar phase at sunset.

Lily of the Valley: Contains powers of the Moon, Venus, and a bit of the Sun. Mostly the plant's roots are used; collect in the Second Quarter close to the Full Moon in the morning.

Linden Tree: Venus, the Sun, and Jupiter. Flowers are picked on the waxing Moon (better right after New Moon) at noon on a sunny day.

Lingonberry (foxberry): Saturn, Jupiter, Mars. Berries are picked in the first lunar quarter and leaves in the second phase, both from sunrise until noon.

Lovage: Contains power of Venus with addition of the Sun and Jupiter. Mostly the roots are used, which should be collected in the end of August in the waning Moon before sunrise.

Male Fern: Contains energies of Uranus, Jupiter, and Mercury. Fern is a magic plant. Picked in the Full Moon on the sixteenth and seventeenth lunar days from sunset till midnight.

Maple: Contains power of Jupiter, the Sun, and Venus. Pick around the Full Moon on the sixteenth and seventeenth lunar days from noon till sunset.

Marshmallow (althaea officialis): As usual, only the root of this plant is used. There are energies of Venus, Jupiter, and Saturn. Picked on the waxing Moon right after sunrise.

Melampyrum Nemorosum: Contains Mercury with the addition of Venus and the Sun. Pick in the Second Quarter before sunrise.

Melissa: This is an herb of Venus and the Sun. Pick on waxing Moon close to the Full Moon at the morning dew.

Mint: Venus, the Sun, and Mercury. Pick in the first lunar phase around sunrise.

Mistletoe (Vescum Album): It has pure Mercury energy. Collect in the Full Moon right after sunset.

Motherwort (Leonurus Cardiaca): A lot of different energies here: Jupiter, Mars, the Sun, and Saturn. Pick on the waxing Moon around noon.

Nettle: This is a magic plant of Mars. Pick from noon until sunset close to the Full Moon. It is better to pick in June after the Sun enters Cancer.

Oak: This is a magic tree of Jupiter. Acorns, buds, and leaves are picked on thirteenth and fourteenth lunar days after sunrise. Oak bark is collected close to the New Moon in the Fourth Quarter before sunset.

Oats: Contains powers of the Sun and Uranus. Gathered in the Third Quarter close to the Full Moon (sixteenth and seventeenth lunar moon days) right after sunset.

Onion: Mars with addition of the Moon and the Sun. Green onions are picked in the waxing Moon from sunrise until noon. The bulbs are gathered in the Full Moon on the sixteenth and seventeenth lunar days around sunset.

Orchis: This is a pure Venus herb. Roots are dug out in the fourth lunar phase around sunset, preferably if the Sun is in Libra.

Oregano: Contains energies of Venus and Mercury. Pick on the waxing Moon after sunrise.

Parsley: Contains powers of Mercury, Jupiter, and Venus. Pick on the thirteenth and fourteenth lunar days at sunset.

Pea: This is a plant of Mercury, Venus, and the Moon. Gather on the thirteenth and fourteenth lunar days in the morning.

Pine: Contains powers of the Sun and Saturn. Cones, needles, and buds are collected in the third lunar phase close to sunset.

Plantago: Contains energies of the Moon, Jupiter, and a little bit of Mercury. Leaves are picked on the waxing Moon at the evening dew, when the plant is blossoming. Roots are dug out in the third lunar phase close to sunset.

Pomegranate: Contains energies of Venus and Jupiter. Picked on the waxing Moon from sunrise unil noon.

Poplar: The Sun and Jupiter. Collect on the waxing Moon at noon.

Potato: Energies of Venus, Jupiter, and the Sun. Harvest on the waning Moon from noon until sunset. Our common potato is also a healing plant, used for body cleansing, toxin removal, and treatment of arthritis.

Primrose: A plant of the Sun and Mercury, it is picked on the waxing Moon at noon.

Pumpkin: Contains the Moon, Mercury, and the Sun. Harvest on the thirteenth and fourteenth lunar days after sunrise.

Purple Marshlocks (Marsh Cinque**foil**): Energies of Mars and the Moon, with the addition of Venus and Mercury. Pick in the second lunar phase (thirteenth to fourteenth lunar days) after sunset.

Radish: Contains energies of Mars, the Moon, and the Sun. Gather around sunset on the thirteenth and fourteenth lunar days.

Raspberry: Energies of Venus, Mercury, and a little bit of Mars. Berries should be picked on the waxing Moon from sunrise until noon, and the leaves in the Second Quarter in the first half of the day. Raspberry roots are dug in the beginning of October before the New Moon (twenty-seventh to thirtieth lunar days) after sunset.

Red Clover: This is a magic herb of Venus. Flowers are picked on the waxing Moon at sunrise. It is better to pick flowers with the left hand. Clover is beneficial for all women. Even taking it like tea might greatly smooth menopause. If it is taken in the special hours its effect will be very strong.

Rhubarb: Contains Jupiter and the Moon. Collect close to the Full Moon (thirteenth and fourteenth lunar days) around sunset.

Rice: Energies of the Sun, Uranus, and Venus. Should be picked in the Second Quarter in the morning.

Rose Hip: Contains Mars, Venus, and Mercury. Collect on the thirteenth and fourteeth lunar days in the morning and after dew.

Rowan: Contains the power of Mars, the Sun, and Jupiter. A variant of blackberries, called Aronia, also has a bit of Saturn. Red rowan berries are picked in the First Quarter before noon. Black Aronia berries are collected in the Second Quarter, from sunrise until sunset.

Salvia (Sage): Contains power of Venus with the addition of Saturn. Picked on the waxing Moon at noon.

Sea-buckthorn: This is a complex plant, containing energies of the Sun, Mars, Jupiter, and the Moon. Picked from noon until sunset in the time of the Full Moon.

Siberian Pine: Jupiter's tree, with very strong energy. Pine cones are collected on the thirteenth and fourteenth lunar days from sunrise until noon.

Silverweed (Argentina Anserina): Mercury, Saturn, the Sun, and Jupiter. Pick in the fourth quarter at noon.

Sorrel (Rumex): Energies of Jupiter, Mercury, and the Moon. Pick in the Second Quarter close to the Full Moon after sunrise.

St.John's Wort: This is a typical Sun herb. Pick in July and August in the first lunar phase between sunrise and noon.

Sunflower: The Sun's plant. Pick at noon right after the New Moon (first, second, and third lunar days). All Sun plants should be collected in quiet, sunny weather.

Tanacetum: Contains energies of the Sun and Uranus. Pick two hours after sunrise or two hours before sunset right after the Full Moon.

Tarragon: It is an herb of Venus, Mercury, and Saturn. Pick on the waxing Moon before sunrise.

Three-lobe Beggarticks: Contains energies of the Sun, Mercury, and a bit of Jupiter. Pick around the Full Moon from noon until sunset.

Thymus: Contains Venus and Mercury. Pick on the waxing Moon at sunrise.

Tomato: The Sun, Mars, and the Moon. If they are picked not just for eating but also for healing purposes, the best time is on the thirteenth and fourteenth lunar days close to sunset.

Valerian: Contains power of Venus and Saturn. The grass is gathered in the First Quarter from noon until sunset; better when the Sun moves from Cancer to Leo. Roots are dug out in the Third Quarter close to sunset.

Viburnum: Energies of Mars, Uranus, and the Moon. Picked in the second lunar phase (better on the thirteenth and fourteenth lunar days) from sunrise until noon.

Violet: This is almost the pure energy of Venus, with a little bit of Mercury. Pick in the Third Quarter close to the Full Moon before sunset.

Water-pepper (persicaria hydropiper): Contains power of Mars and the Moon. This herb is picked in the Second Quarter before sunrise.

White Acacia: Contains power of Venus, the Moon, Jupiter, and Mars. Flowers are collected in the first or second lunar phases from sunrise until noon. Acacia's pods are gathered in the third phase, also from sunrise until noon.

Willow: This is one of the Moon's trees, with the addition of Saturn. Branches and leaves are gathered on the waxing Moon from sunrise until noon.

Wormwood: This is a complex plant: Mars, Neptune, the Sun, and Jupiter. Picked on the waning Moon after sunset.

Yarrow: Contains power of Uranus, the Moon, and Saturn. Picked in the fourth lunar phase close to sunset. The Sun should be in Leo and the weather sunny and quiet.

Yellow Melilot (Yellow Sweet Clover): The Sun and Mercury. Gather in the First Quarter around noon.

Zucchini: Contains power of Mercury, the Moon, the Sun, and Jupiter. Collect on the waxing Moon in the morning (before noon).

In the list above you can see the ideal conditions for picking specific herbs. However, you can't always follow all of them because of the weather, for example, or urgency. In this case, follow this general rule: above-ground parts of plants should be picked on the waxing Moon; roots should be dug out on the waning Moon, preferably in the fourth quarter.

It makes sense to also take the days of the week into consideration. Monday is ruled by the Moon, Tuesday by Mars, Wednesday by Mercury, Thursday by Jupiter, Friday by Venus, Saturday by Saturn, and Sunday by the Sun. It is best to pick the plant on the day that is ruled by the planet that is also the ruler of the plant. For example, when I needed a plant of Venus in order to block a nephritic colic, I searched for lilac flowers on a Friday on the waxing Moon in the first half of the day (ideally it should be done at sunrise).

Once you have gathered the herbs, the next step will be to figure out when decoction (or tincture) should be prepared and then taken.

Time for Taking Herbs

Medicine should be taken in the hours of the planet relative to the organ being treated. Finding planetary hours isn't as simple as you might expect. In this case one hour equals 60 minutes only in days of vernal and autumnal equinox. In other instances, hours have different lengths depending on the durations of day and night.

The seven-pointed Star of Magus determines the planetary hours (Figure 17). This star is based on the Chaldean Row, which was brought to Europe from Babylon. The information given by the Star of Magus is universal: it was used in Egypt and ancient India and is also related to Cabbala. The Star of Magus contains seven main planets in a particular order: Mars, the Sun, Venus, Mercury, the Moon, Saturn, and Jupiter. Every astrological day begins from sunrise. The planet of the first hour is the planet that rules the day of the week. For example: the Sun for Sunday or Mars for Tuesday.

We assume that a day has twelve hours and a night has twelve hours, but these are not standard, sixty-minute hours. First the duration of day and night needs to be found. Day is the interval between sunrise and sunset; night is the period between sunset and sunrise of the next day. Let's take June 28, 2010 as an example (not a leap year). Sunrise was at 5:16 a.m., sunset at 9:15 p.m., and sunrise of the next day at 5:17 a.m. The duration of the day was thus 959 minutes and the night was 482 minutes. Dividing these numbers by 12 we get: one daytime hour lasts 79.92 minutes and one night hour 40.17 minutes.

Because June 28, 2010, was Monday, the first hour was an hour of the Moon. It lasted from 5:16 until 6:36 a.m. The next hour was an hour of Saturn and lasted from 6:36 until 7:56 a.m., followed by an hour of Jupiter and so on. From sunset the hour of Venus began and lasted from 9:15 until 9:55 p.m. (only 40 minutes).

Some astrological software provides planetary hours.

What about planets of the higher octave? They are not forgotten. There is a so-called "higher week" where Tuesday starts with Pluto's hour; Wednesday, Uranus; Thursday, Chiron; Friday, Neptune; and Saturday, Proserpina. You can find the rulers of the hours in Appendix 3.

It is also better to prepare decoctions in the hours of the planet that is the ruler of the organ to be healed; in this way the proper rhythm will be maintained. Planetary hours repeat three times a day. However, when they occur late at night it doesn't make sense to wake a patient to take medication. Because it is better to take decoctions three or four times a day, it is useful to know that it can be also done in the hours of the Sun, the Moon, and Mercury if they are positive. Hours of a Hyleg planet are also good. It is pointless to take herbs in the hours of Antihyleg and malicious planets.

Diet and Lifestyle Recommendations

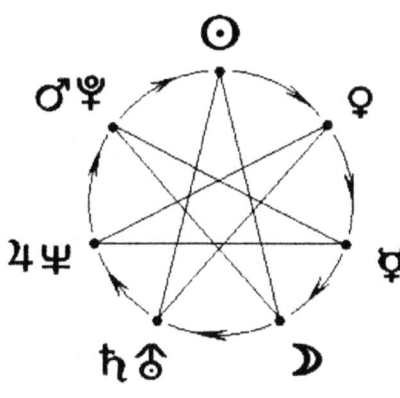

Figure 17. The Star of Magus.

It is possible to give some recommendation about diet based on the element predominant in the chart. Pay attention that "predominant element" doesn't necessarily mean the element of the birth sign. If the birth Sun is in Taurus it doesn't necessarily mean that the most prominent element is earth. There could be a planetary gathering in Gemini, so the main element would be air. It is necessary to look at the signs of all twelve planets.

There is a simple method for calculating the power of elements. Each planet is given a certain point value according to its importance. The Sun and the Moon, being luminaries, will have 2 points. Other personal planets (Mercury, Venus, and Mars) are given 1.5 points. All other planets are given 1 point. To determine the power of elements we consider all of the planets that are located in their signs. For example, Venus and Mercury are in Gemini, Saturn in Aquarius and Proserpina in Libra.

1.5 + 1.5 + 1 +1 = 5. Air has 5 points.

Sometimes none of the elements is very prominent. In order to be the main element it has to be significantly stronger than the others (typically 1.5 times). For instance, fire has 1.5 points; air, 4; earth, 2.5; and water, 7.5. It is clear here that water is the predominant element. Another example: if we have fire at 3.5 points, air at 4, earth at 5 and water at 3, we are dealing with a horoscope of mixed elements.

Recommendations given below concern only charts with predominant elements.

Water: People with the dominant element of water need good nutrition in the third lunar phase, although they shouldn't eat much in the first one. In the fourth lunar phase these people should be quite picky about what they eat and it is better to exclude heavy food (meat, mushrooms) and salty products in this lunar quarter. It is also good to limit consumption of white bread, tea, coffee, onions, and garlic. Vegetables and fruits are beneficial (especially sweet fruits and berries), as are juices.

Because of the extreme sensitivity of the water element it is better not to participate in any group practices in the fourth phase of the Moon. Group practices here refer to meditation, psychological workshops, etc.

Fire: For people with a strong fire element, it isn't recommended that they eat a lot in the morning. The maximum amount of food should be consumed between noon and 2:00 p.m. It is good to eat more in the third lunar phase and less in the first.

Ensure there is enough protein in the diet. It is good to eat more grains, greens, fruits, and berries. It is better not to mix protein with carbohydrates. No deep-fried foods. Fats should be in the diet, but it would be best if they are from vegetable oils.

Sweets, tea, and coffee should be limited. Green tea is healthier.

For prevention and treatment of illnesses, fire people can use breathing practices. The best time for this kind of exercise is at sunrise or sunset. If they decide to take a course of herbal treatment, it is better to do so at the same time (sunrise, sunset). Some people with a strong fire element have difficulties keeping good intentions for a lengthy time period and tend to give up. Those in this category can achieve more success by planning any kind of activity for just one lunar phase, with the first one preferably starting from the New Moon.

Air: People of the air element should have a sufficient meal in the morning, between 8:00 and 10:00 a.m. It isn't useful to eat after sunset. They can eat a lot in the fourth lunar phase and less in the second one. The third lunar phase is the phase of air. In this time it is better not to eat much in the way of "light" food (veggies, fruits) because there might be too much of this element. It is helpful to eat dairy products in the third phase and to drink a lot of liquids.

These people can eat sour products, but they should refrain from bitter ones. Sweet and salty are neutral for air. Coffee, potatoes, mushrooms, and vegetables ruled by the Moon (e.g., cucumbers, zucchini, pumpkin) shouldn't be consumed in large amounts.

In the third lunar phase it is beneficial to try to improve health using herbal treatments. Water treatments are also good for air people.

Earth: The right diet for those of the earth element is more important than for any other element because earth is connected with the assimilation and transformation of the matter the human organism consumes. Virgos should take the matter of nutrition especially seriously.

Earth people should follow an even schedule of taking meals: in the morning around 7:00 to 8:00 a.m., again at noon and in the evening before sunset. For them it is better to eat more in the first lunar phase and less in the third. It is good to limit butter, milk, white bread, sweets, and salt. Other dairy products are useful (yogurt, kefir), as are sweet fruits, berries, and all vegetables.

Information for Energy Healers

Influences on one's aura can cure and even prevent illness. I won't go deeply into aspects of energy healing, although I have practiced it successfully for a long time. Because this book is astrological in its focus, I'll give a few recommendations to healers from the astrological point of view.

Who can be a healer and what kind of patients can he or she work with? Can anyone practice energy healing? Unfortunately, the answer is no. In this matter we have to be careful in order not to harm our patients and even ourselves. What might be in a chart that would indicate a person is capable of working with energies? First of all are the aspects from higher planets (Uranus, Pluto, and Neptune) to the Sun and the Moon. Mars should be also taken into consideration.

Second, it is necessary to know the main element. People with strong fire and water in their charts are considered the best healers. They possess the powerful energy of fire and subconsciously tune in to the cosmic rhythms peculiar to the water element. These people can always feel who they can treat and when to do it without looking at the astrological calendar.

It is necessary for people with the pure water element to have a strong Mars or Sun in the natal chart. They can easily feel a patient and are very sensitive to his or her problems (sometimes too sensitive). Water healers can easily expend their energy or, moreover, catch something bad from the patient. Healers of this category must regularly perform protective and cleansing practices.

People of the fire element with prominent Neptune are good healers. People with the predominant earth element have a greatly reduced chance of being successful in this area. With certain strong aspects they nevertheless can work with energies even though they usually are not able to feel subtle energy. They might work much better with massage.

People with an air or air and water horoscope probably should avoid practicing healing. They can be excellent mediums but it is difficult for them to work with energies because there is no stability and they easily absorb unwanted energy. However, those in this category make the best patients; it is easy to work with them.

It is also helpful to know what element predominates in the patient's chart. Healers of fire signs treat well people of the earth element, but not so well patients of the water element. On the other side, the rare earth healers are excellent when it comes to curing patients of fire signs. However, it is difficult for them to sense air people.

So, fire and earth can treat each other, and air and water are good in cooperation. As mentioned above, healers with strong fire and water in their charts can treat anyone.

At a young age I couldn't see my own abilities in energy healing. I have a predominant water element with the addition of earth and was sure I simply didn't have enough strength to do this. (It is difficult to be unbiased about your own chart.) In looking at my own horoscope I didn't notice a sextile between Uranus and the Moon, a Neptune trine with the Sun, Pluto-Sun sextile, Pluto-Mars trine, and some others. With time they showed themselves and it turned out that I am able to see with my hands (as well as traditional diagnostic tools) and also to heal. However, if my water element didn't have support from strong planets, patients would have consumed me in a split second. The protection code was very useful here as well.

When it comes to the time for healing practices each of us has to find the proper time by paying attention to our intuition. It is good to look at the calendar of moon days and exclude some of them; for example, the ninth and twenty-ninth lunar days. It is also considered inadvisable to heal in the hours of Pluto because its very strong energy flows become apparent, blocking any individual energy influences.

Before concluding I would like to share some more information with energy healers who work with chakras. Reiki practitioners can also adapt this information for their needs.

If you have a chance to see a patient's medical chart and figure out the Hyleg and Antihyleg planets, your healing work will be more efficient. We always start with the Hyleg because the first task is to give energy to the sick person. Energizing the chakra related to the Hyleg planet can help the recovery process.

- Muladhara, the Root Chakra: Saturn
- Swadhisthana, the Sacral Charka: Jupiter
- Manipura, the Solar Plexus: Mars
- Anahata, the Heart Chakra: Venus
- Vishudha, the Throat Chakra: Mercury
- Ajna, the Brow Chakra: Moon
- Sahasrara, the Crown Chakra: Sun

When you pump energy to the Hyleg's chakra, be extra careful with two top chakras: Ajna and Sahasrara. Don't give too much! In this case less is better than more. Too much energy given to a person who isn't ready can cause additional health problems.

The Antihyleg's chakra needs a lot of cleansing, not only through energy work but also via patient's spiritual development.

I wish you all luck in your noble work.

Namaste.

Medical Glossary

Adrenal Glands: endocrine glands situated above the kidneys.

Alzheimer's Disease: gradual shrinking of the brain where the nerve fibers become tangled resulting in a progressive decline in mental activities.

Anemia: a decrease in the production of red blood cells and/or haemoglobin. This may be caused by excessive blood loss reducing the amount of red blood cells in the body, lack of iron affecting the haemoglobin function, or dysfunction in the bone marrow resulting in loss of production of new blood cells.

Angina: a chest pain due in general to obstruction or spasm of the coronary arteries.

Arterial Thrombosis: clotting of blood in an artery obstructing normal blood flow.

Arteriosclerosis: the walls of the arteries lose their elasticity and harden. This has the effect of raising the blood pressure.

Arthritis: inflammation of the joints. Arthritis can be acute or chronic.

Asthma: difficulty in breathing caused by narrowing of the airways. It may be triggered by external factors, known as extrinsic asthma, or internal factors, known as intrinsic asthma.

Atherosclerosis: a narrowing of the arteries caused by a buildup of fats, including cholesterol.

Atrophy: wasting of muscle tissue.

Bechterew's Disease: a chronic inflammatory disease of an axial skeleton that can cause eventual fusion of the spine.

Bronchitis: inflammation of the lining of the bronchi.

Cataract: a clouding of the lens inside the eye that leads to a decrease of vision.

Cerebral Palsy: a permanent disorder of the brain affecting the control of muscles. Muscles have reduced control and go into spasms.

Cirrhosis of the Liver: hardening of the liver generally caused by the consumption of excessive amounts of alcohol.

Cholecystitis: inflammation of the gall-bladder that occurs most commonly due to obstruction of the cystic duct with the gallstones.

Colitis: an inflammation of the large intestine resulting in diarrhea that is then combined with blood and mucus as a result of damage to the intestinal lining.

Coronary Thrombosis: a common cause of heart attack where an artery supplying the heart is obstructed.

Cramp: a sudden involuntary contraction of a muscle causing acute pain.

Diabetes: a condition whereby the body cannot use the sugars and carbohydrates from the diet. The hormone insulin, which is produced by the pancreas, helps to regulate the use of sugars by the body. Diabetes occurs when the pancreas fails to produce enough insulin, resulting in a build-up of sugar in the blood.

Fibroids: non-cancerous growths which develop in the walls of the uterus.

Emphysema: inflammation of the alveoli in the lungs causing reduced blood flow through the lungs. It is usually associated with bronchitis and/or old age.

Gastritis: irritation or inflammation of the stomach. Can be associated with something that has been eaten or drunk.

Glaucoma: optic nerve damage due to the ocular hypertension (increased fluid pressure in the eye).

Hemophilia: the blood is unable to clot, resulting in excessive blood loss.

Hepatitis: inflammation of the liver caused by different viruses that are transmitted by infected blood.

Hypertension: high blood pressure.

Hypotension: low blood pressure.

Laryngitis: inflammation of the larynx producing hoarseness and/or loss of voice.

Leukemia: over-production of white blood cells resulting in cancer of the blood.

Meningitis: a severe infection of the membrane surrounding the brain and spinal cord.

Muscular Dystrophies: genetic diseases resulting in the collapse of muscle leading to loss of function.

Myoma: tumor composed of muscular tissue.

Neuralgia: pressure on a nerve caused by irritation. Pain can be felt along the length of the nerve as well as at the point of pressure.

Neurodermatitis: a skin disorder characterized by chronic itching and scratching.

Oedema: swelling caused by excess fluid from the circulatory system that has accumulated within the tissues.

Osteochondritis: softening of bone causing the bone to change shape and become deformed.

Peritonitis: an inflammation of the peritoneum, the thin tissue that lines the inner wall of the abdomen and covers most of the abdominal organs.

Pharyngitis: inflammation of the pharynx resulting in a sore throat and may be either acute or chronic.

Piles (Hemorroids): swollen veins in the anus causing pain and discomfort. Bleeding from these veins can result in anaemia due to the excessive loss of iron in the blood.

Pneumonia: inflammation of the lungs from either a bacterial or viral infection that results in chest pain, dry cough, fever etc. Bacterial pneumonia tends to last longer.

Pyelonephritis: inflammation of the kidneys due to an infection.

Rhinitis: inflammation of the mucous lining of the nasal cavity causing a blocked, runny and stuffy nose.

Sinusitis: inflammation of the mucous lining of the sinuses causing a blockage that can be very painful, swollen, and sore. It can be acute, usually accompanying a cold, or chronic when there are recurrent blockages.

Spasm: a sudden, involuntary muscle contraction.

Stroke: a sudden loss of function on one side of the body caused by an interruption of the blood supply to part of the brain.

Tachycardia: an increased heart rate.

Thrombophlebitis: inflammation of a section of a vein usually occurring in the legs.

Thrombus: a blood clot in the blood vessels or the heart.

Varicose Veins: ineffective valves in veins that cause the blood to collect in the veins instead of returning to the heart. This results in veins becoming distended and painful.

Ulcer: a break in the surface of any part of the body. Commonly associated with various parts of the digestive system where there is a break in the lining of the alimentary canal caused by the over-production of acid in the gastric and intestinal juices.

Appendix 1. Ephemeris of Proserpina

Note: The degrees, minutes, and seconds listed below are written in this form: 7.47.56, which equates to 7°47'56".

Proserpina in Libra

1935

January	7.44.59R	May	7.18.38	September	7.52.01
February	7.38.12	June	7.20.19D	October	8.04.02
March	7.29.40	July	7.27.30	November	8.12.19
April	7.22.16	August	7.38.52	December	8.15.17

1936

January	8.12.45R	May	7.46.20	September	8.19.30
February	8.06.01	June	7.47.56D	October	8.31.33
March	7.57.29	July	7.55.02	November	8.39.55
April	7.50.03	August	8.06.22	December	8.42.58

1937

January	8.40.31R	May	8.14.02	September	8.46.59
February	8.33.49	June	8.15.33D	October	8.59.04
March	8.25. 17	July	8.22.34	November	9.07.30
April	8.17.49	August	8.33.51	December	9.10.38

1938

January	9.08.16R	May	8.41.44	September	9.14.28
February	9.01.37	June	8.43.10D	October	9.26.35
March	8.53.06	July	8.50.06	November	9.35.06
April	8.45.36	August	9.01.20	December	9.38.19

1939

January	9.36.01R	May	9.09.27	September	9.47.57
February	9.29.26	June	9.10.47D	October	9.54.06
March	9.20.55	July	9.17.39	November	10.02.41
April	9.13.23	August	9.28.50	December	10.06.00

1940

January	10.03.47R	May	9.37.09	September	10.09.25
February	9.57.14	June	9.38.24D	October	10.21.37
March	9.48.44	July	9.45.11	November	10.30.16
April	9.41.09	August	9.56.19	December	10.33.40

1941

January	10.31.32R	May	10.04.51	September	10.36.54
February	10.23.03	June	10.06.01D	October	10.49.08
March	10.16.33	July	10.12.44	November	10.57.52
April	10.08.56	August	10.23.48	December	11.01.21

1942

January	10.59.17R	May	10.32.34	September	11.04.23
February	10.52.51	June	10.33.38D	October	11.16.39
March	10.44.22	July	10.40.16	November	11.25.27
April	10.36.43	August	10.51.18	December	11.29.01

1943

January	11.27.03R	May	11.00.17	September	11.31.52
February	11.20.39	June	11.01.16D	October	11.44.10
March	11.12.11	July	11.07.49	November	11.53.02
April	11.04.30	August	11.18.47	December	11.56.41

1944

January	11.54.48R	May	11.27.59	September	11.59.21
February	11.48.28	June	11.28.53D	October	12.11.41
March	11.40.00	July	11.35.21	November	12.20.37
April	11.32.17	August	11.46.17	December	12.24.22

1945

January	12.22.33R	May	11.55.42	September	12.26.50
February	12.16.16	June	11.56.31D	October	12.39.12
March	12.07.49	July	12.02.54	November	12.48.12
April	12.00.04	August	12.13.46	December	12.52.02

1946

January	12.50.18R	May	12.23.25	September	12.54.18
February	12.44.04	June	12.24.09D	October	13.06.43
March	12.35.37	July	12.30.27	November	13.15.47
April	12.27.51	August	12.41.16	December	13.19.42

1947

January	13.18.03R	May	12.51.08	September	13.21.47
February	13.11.52	June	12.51.46D	October	13.34.13
March	13.03.26	July	12.58.00	November	13.43.21
April	12.55.38	August	13.08.45	December	13.47.22

1948

January	13.45.48R	May	13.18.51	September	13.49.16
February	13.39.40	June	13.19.24D	October	14.01.44
March	13.31.15	July	13.25.33	November	14.10.56
April	13.23.25	August	13.36.15	December	14.15.02

1949

January	14.13.32R	May	13.46.34	September	14.16.45
February	14.07.28	June	13.47.02D	October	14.29.15
March	13.59.04	July	13.53.06	November	14.38.31
April	13.51.12	August	14.03.45	December	14.42.41

1950

January	14.41.17R	May	14.14.17	September	14.44.14
February	14.35.17	June	14.14.40D	October	14.56.45
March	14.26.53	July	14.20.39	November	15.06.05
April	14.18.59	August	14.31.14	December	15.10.21

1951

January	15.09.02R	May	14.42.00	September	15.11.42
February	15.03.05	June	14.42.18D	October	15.24.16
March	14.54.42	July	14.48.12	November	15.33.40
April	14.46.46	August	14.58.44	December	15.38.01

1952

January	15.26.46R	May	15.09.44	September	15.39.11
February	15.30.53	June	15.09.56R	October	15.51.46
March	15.22.31	July	15.15.45	November	16.01.14
April	15.14.33	August	15.26.14	December	16.15.40

1953

January	16.04.31R	May	15.37.27	September	16.06.40
February	15.58.41	June	15.37.35D	October	16.19.17
March	15.50.20	July	15.43.18	November	16.28.49
April	15.42.21	August	15.53.44	December	16.33.20

1954

January	16.32.15R	May	16.05.10	September	16.34.09
February	16.26.28	June	16.05.13D	October	16.46.17
March	16.18.09	July	16.10.52	November	16.56.33
April	16.10.08	August	16.21.13	December	17.00.59

1955

January	17.00.00R	May	16.32.54	September	17.01.37
February	16.54.16	June	16.32.51D	October	17.14.17
March	16.45.58	July	16.38.25	November	17.23.57
April	16.37.55	August	16.48.43	December	17.28.39

1956

January	17.27.44R	May	17.00.38	September	17.29.06
February	17.22.04	June	17.00.30D	October	17.41.48
March	17.13.47	July	17.05.59	November	17.51.31
April	17.05.43	August	17.16.13	December	17.56.18

1957

January	17.55.28R	May	17.28.21	September	17.56.35
February	17.49.52	June	17.28.08D	October	18.09.18
March	17.41.36	July	17.33.32	November	18.19.05
April	17.33.30	August	17.43.43	December	18.23.57

1958

January	18.23.12R	May	17.56.05	September	18.24.04
February	18.17.40	June	17.55.47D	October	18.36.48
March	18.09.25	July	18.01.06	November	18.46.39
April	18.01.18	August	18.11.13	December	18.51.36

1959

January	18.50.56R	May	18.23.49	September	18.51.32
February	18.45.28	June	18.23.26D	October	19.04.18
March	18.37.14	July	18.28.40	November	19.14.13
April	18.29.06	August	18.38.43	December	19.19.15

1960

January	19.18.41R	May	18.51.33	September	19.19.01
February	19.13.15	June	18.51.05D	October	19.31.48
March	19.05.03	July	18.56.13	November	19.41.47
April	18.56.53	August	19.06.13	December	19.46.54

1961

January	19.46.25R	May	19.19.17	September	19.46.30
February	19.41.03	June	19.18.43D	October	19.59.19
March	19.32.52	July	19.23.47	November	20.09.21
April	19.24.41	August	19.33.43	December	20.14.33

1962

January	20.14.08R	May	19.47.01	September	20.13.59
February	20.08.51	June	19.46.22D	October	20.26.49
March	20.00.41	July	19.51.21	November	20.36.55
April	19.52.28	August	20.01.14	December	20.42.12

1963

January	20.41.52R	May	20.14.45	September	20.41.27
February	20.36.38	June	20.14.01D	October	20.54.19
March	20.28.30	July	20.18.55	November	21.04.28
April	20.20.16	August	20.28.44	December	21.09.50

1964

January	21.09.36R	May	20.42.29	September	21.08.56
February	21.04.26	June	20.41.41D	October	21.21.49
March	20.56.19	July	20.46.29	November	21.30.02
April	20.48.04	August	20.56.14	December	21.37.29

1965

January	21.37.20R	May	21.10.13	September	21.36.25
February	21.32.13	June	21.09.20D	October	21.49.19
March	21.24.08	July	21.14.03	November	21.59.35
April	21.15.52	August	21.23.44	December	22.05.07

1966

January	22.05.03R	May	21.37.57	September	22.03.54
February	22.00.01	June	21.36.59D	October	22.16.48
March	21.51.57	July	21.41.37	November	22.27.09
April	21.43.40	August	21.51.15	December	22.32.46

1967

January	22.32.47D	May	22.05.42	September	22.31.22
February	22.27.48	June	22.04.38D	October	22.44.18
March	22.19.46	July	22.09.12	November	22.54.42
April	22.11.28	August	22.18.45	December	23.00.24

1968

January	23.00.30R	May	22.33.26	September	22.58.51
February	22.55.36	June	22.32.18D	October	23.11.48
March	22.47.35	July	22.36.46	November	23.22.15
April	22.39.16	August	22.46.15	December	23.28.02

1969

January	23.28.14R	May	23.01.11	September	23.26.20
February	23.23.23	June	22.59.57D	October	23.39.18
March	23.15.24	July	23.04.20	November	23.49.49
April	23.07.03	August	23.13.46	December	23.55.41

1970

January	23.55.57R	May	23.28.55	September	23.53.49
February	23.51.10	June	23.27.37D	October	24.06.48
March	23.43.13	July	23.31.55	November	24.17.22
April	23.34.51	August	23.41.16	December	24.23.19

1971

January	24.23.40R	May	23.56.40	September	24.21.17
February	24.18.57	June	23.55.17D	October	24.34.17
March	24.11.02	July	23.59.29	November	24.44.55
April	24.02.40	August	24.08.47	December	24.50.57

1972

January	24.51.23R	May	24.24.25	September	24.48.46
February	24.46.45	June	24.22.57D	October	25.01.47
March	24.38.51	July	24.27.04	November	25.12.28
April	24.30.28	August	24.36.17	December	25.18.25

1973

January	25.19.07R	May	24.52.09	September	25.16.15
February	25.14.32	June	24.50.36D	October	25.29.17
March	25.06.40	July	24.54.39	November	25.40.01
April	24.58.16	August	25.03.48	December	25.46.12

1974

January	25.46.50R	May	25.19.54	September	25.43.44
February	25.42.19	June	25.18.16D	October	25.56.46
March	25.34.29	July	25.22.13	November	26.07.34
April	25.26.40	August	25.31.19	December	26.13.50

1975

January	26.14.33R	May	25.47.39	September	26.11.13
February	26.10.06	June	25.45.56D	October	26.24.16
March	26.02.18	July	25.49.48	November	26.35.07
April	25.53.52	August	25.58.50	December	26.41.28

1976

January	26.42.15R	May	26.15.24	September	26.38.40
February	26.37.53	June	26.13.37D	October	26.51.45
March	26.30.07	July	26.17.23	November	27.02.39
April	26.21.40	August	26.26.20	December	27.09.06

1977

January	27.09.58R	May	26.43.09	September	27.06.10
February	27.05.40	June	26.41.17D	October	27.19.15
March	26.57.56	July	26.44.58	November	27.30.12
April	26.49.28	August	26.53.51	December	27.36.43]

1978

January	27.37.41R	May	27.10.54	September	27.33.39
February	27.33.27	June	27.08.57D	October	27.46.44
March	27.25.45	July	27.12.33	November	27.57.45
April	27.17.17	August	27.21.22	December	28.04.21

1979

January	28.05.24R	May	27.38.39	September	28.01.08
February	28.01.13	June	27.36.37D	October	28.14.14
March	27.53.34	July	27.40.08	November	28.25.17
April	27.45.05	August	27.48.53	December	28.31.58

1980

January	28.33.06R	May	28.06.25	September	28.28.37
February	28.29.00	June	28.04.18D	October	28.41.43
March	28.21.23	July	28.07.44	November	28.52.50
April	28.12.53	August	28.16.24	December	28.59.35

1981

January	29.00.49	May	28.34.40	September	28.56.06
February	28.56.47	June	28.31.58D	October	29.09.13
March	28.49.12	July	28.35.19	November	29.20.22
April	28.40.42	August	28.43.55	December	29.27.12

1982

January	29.28.31R	May	29.01.55	September	29.23.35
February	29.24.34	June	28.59.39D	October	29.36.42
March	29.17.01	July	29.02.54	November	29.47.55
April	29.08.30	August	29.11.26	December	29.54.50

1983

January	29.56.13R	May	29.29.41	September	29.51.04
February	29.52.20	June	29.27.20D	October	0.04.11(Scor)
March	29.44.50	July	29.30.30	November	0.15.27
April	29.36.18	August	29.38.57	December	0.22.27

Proserpina in Scorpio

1984

January	0.23.56R	May	29.57.26 (Lib)	September	0.18.32
February	0.20.07	June	29.55.00D	October	0.31.41
March	0.12.38	July	29.58.05	November	0.42.59
April	0.04.07	August	0.06.28 (Scor)	December	0.50.04

1985

January	0.51.38R	May	0.25.12	September	0.46.01
February	0.47.53	June	0.22.41D	October	0.59.10
March	0.40.27	July	0.25.41	November	1.10.31
April	0.31.55	August	0.34.00	December	1.17.40

1986

January	1.19.20R	May	0.52.57	September	1.13.30
February	1.15.40	June	0.50.22D	October	1.26.29
March	1.08.16	July	0.53.16	November	1.38.03
April	0.59.44	August	1.01.31	December	1.45.17

1987

January	1.47.02R	May	1.20.43	September	1.40.59
February	1.43.26	June	1.18.03D	October	1.54.08
March	1.36.05	July	1.20.52	November	2.05.36
April	1.37.32	August	1.29.02	December	2.12.54

1988

January	2.14.44R	May	1.48.29	September	2.08.28
February	2.11.13	June	1.45.44	October	2.21.38
March	2.03.54	July	1.48.28D	November	2.33.08
April	1.55.21	August	1.56.34	December	2.40.31

1989

January	2.42.26R	May	2.16.14	September	2.35.57
February	2.38.59	June	2.13.25	October	2.49.07
March	2.31.42	July	2.16.04D	November	3.00.39
April	2.23.10	August	2.24.05	December	3.08.07

1990

January	3.10.08R	May	2.44.00	September	3.03.26
February	3.06.45	June	2.41.06	October	3.16.36
March	2.59.31	July	2.43.40D	November	3.28.11
April	2.50.58	August	2.51.37	December	3.35.44

1991

January	3.37.49R	May	3.11.46	September	3.30.55
February	3.34.33	June	3.08.48	October	3.44.05
March	3.27.20	July	3.11.16D	November	3.55.43
April	3.18.47	August	3.19.08	December	4.03.20

1992

January	4.05.31R	May	3.39.32	September	3.58.24
February	4.02.18	June	3.36.29	October	4.11.34
March	3.55.09	July	3.38.52D	November	4.23.15
April	3.46.35	August	3.46.40	December	4.30.57

1993

January	4.33.13R	May	4.07.18	September	4.25.53
February	4.30.04	June	4.04.11	October	4.39.03
March	4.22.57	July	4.06.28D	November	4.50.47
April	4.14.24	August	4.14.12	December	4.58.33

1994

January	5.00.54R	May	4.35.04	September	4.53.23
February	4.57.50	June	4.31.52	October	5.06.32
March	4.50.46	July	4.34.05D	November	5.18.18
April	4.42.13	August	4.41.43	December	5.26.09

1995

January	5.28.35R	May	5.02.50	September	5.20.52
February	5.25.36	June	4.59.34	October	5.34.01
March	5.18.35	July	5.01.41D	November	5.45.50
April	5.10.01	August	5.09.15	December	5.53.45

1996

January	5.56.17R	May	5.30.37	September	5.48.21
February	5.53.22	June	5.27.16	October	6.01.30
March	5.46.23	July	5.29.18D	November	6.13.21
April	5.37.50	August	5.36.47	December	6.21.21

1997

January	6.23.58R	May	5.58.23	September	6.15.50
February	6.21.08	June	5.54.57	October	6.28.59
March	6.14.12	July	5.2654D	November	6.40.53
April	6.05.39	August	6.04.19	December	6.48.57

1998

January	6.51.39R	May	6.26.09	September	6.43.19
February	6.48.53	June	6.22.39	October	6.56.28
March	6.42.00	July	6.24.31D	November	7.08.24
April	6.33.28	August	6.31.51	December	7.16.33

1999

January	7.19.20	May	6.53.56	September	7.10.48
February	7.16.39R	June	6.50.21	October	7.23.57
March	7.09.49	July	6.52.07D	November	7.35.56
April	7.01.16	August	6.59.23	December	7.44.09

2000

January	7.47.01	May	7.21.42	September	7.38.18
February	7.44.25R	June	7.18.03	October	7.51.26
March	7.37.37	July	7.19.44D	November	8.03.27
April	7.29.05	August	7.26.55	December	8.11.44

2001

January	8.14.42	May	7.49.28	September	8.05.47
February	8.12.10R	June	7.45.45	October	8.18.55
March	8.05.26	July	7.47.21D	November	8.30.58
April	7.56.54	August	7.54.27	December	8.39.20

2002

January	8.42.23	May	8.17.15	September	8.33.16
February	8.39.56R	June	8.13.27	October	8.46.24
March	8.33.14	July	8.14.58D	November	8.58.20
April	8.24.43	August	8.22.00	December	9.06.56

2003

January	9.10.04	May	8.45.01	September	9.00.46
February	9.07.41R	June	8.41.10	October	9.13.53
March	9.01.03	July	8.42.35D	November	9.26.01
April	8.52.32	August	8.49.32	December	9.34.31

2004

January	9.37.45	May	9.12.48	September	9.28.15
February	9.35.27R	June	9.08.52	October	9.41.22
March	9.28.51	July	9.01.12D	November	9.53.32
April	9.20.21	August	9.17.04	December	10.02.06

2005

January	10.05.25	May	9.40.35	September	9.55.44
February	10.03.12R	June	9.36.34	October	10.08.51
March	9.56.40	July	9.37.49D	November	10.21.03
April	9.48.09	August	9.44.37	December	10.29.43

2006

January	10.33.06	May	10.08.22	September	10.23.14
February	10.30.58R	June	10.04.17	October	10.36.20
March	10.24.28	July	10.05.27D	November	10.48.34
April	10.15.58	August	10.12.09	December	10.57.17

2007

January	11.00.46	May	10.36.08	September	10.50.43
February	10.58.43R	June	10.31.59	October	11.03.49
March	10.52.16	July	10.33.04D	November	11.16.05
April	10.43.47	August	10.39.42	December	11.24.52

2008

January	11.28.37	May	11.03.55	September	11.18.13
February	11.26.28R	June	10.59.42	October	11.31.17
March	11.20.05	July	11.00.41D	November	11.43.36
April	11.11.36	August	11.07.14	December	11.52.27

2009

January	11.56.07	May	11.31.42	September	11.45.52
February	11.54.13R	June	11.27.25	October	11.58.46
March	11.47.53	July	11.28.19D	November	12.11.07
April	11.39.25	August	11.34.47	December	12.20.02

2010

January	12.23.47	May	11.59.29	September	12.13.12
February	12.21.58R	June	11.55.08	October	12.26.15
March	12.15.41	July	11.55.56D	November	12.38.37
April	12.07.14	August	12.02.20	December	12.47.37

2011

January	12.51.27	May	12.27.16	September	12.40.41
February	12.49.43R	June	12.22.50	October	12.53.44
March	12.43.29	July	12.23.34D	November	13.06.08
April	12.35.03	August	12.29.52	December	13.15.12

2012

January	13.19.07	May	12.55.03	September	13.08.11
February	13.17.28R	June	12.50.33	October	13.21.13
March	13.11.18	July	12.51.12D	November	13.33.29
April	13.02.52	August	12.57.25	December	13.42.47

2013

January	13.46.47	May	13.22.50	September	13.35.40
February	13.45.13R	June	13.18.16	October	13.48.41
March	13.39.06	July	13.18.50D	November	14.01.10
April	13.30.41	August	13.24.58	December	14.10.22

2014

January	14.14.27	May	13.50.37	September	14.03.10
February	14.12.58R	June	13.45.59	October	14.16.10
March	14.06.54	July	13.46.28D	November	14.28.40
April	13.58.30	August	13.52.31	December	14.37.56

2015

January	14.42.07	May	14.18.24	September	14.30.40
February	14.40.42R	June	14.13.43	October	14.43.39
March	14.34.42	July	14.14.06D	November	14.56.11
April	14.26.19	August	14.20.04	December	15.05.31

2016

January	15.09.47	May	14.46.12	September	14.58.10
February	15.08.27R	June	14.41.26	October	15.11.08
March	15.02.30	July	14.41.44D	November	15.23.41
April	14.54.08	August	14.47.37	December	15.33.05

2017

January	15.37.26	May	15.13.59	September	15.25.39
February	15.36.12R	June	15.09.09	October	15.38.37
March	15.30.18	July	15.09.22D	November	15.51.12
April	15.21.57	August	15.15.11	December	16.00.40

2018

January	16.05.06	May	15.41.46	September	15.53.09
February	16.03.56R	June	15.36.52	October	16.06.05
March	15.58.06	July	15.37.00D	November	16.18.42
April	15.49.46	August	15.42.44	December	16.28.14

2019

January	16.32.45	May	16.09.34	September	16.20.39
February	16.31.41R	June	16.04.36	October	16.33.34
March	16.25.54	July	16.04.38D	November	16.46.13
April	16.17.35	August	16.10.17	December	16.55.48

2020

January	17.00.25	May	16.37.21	September	16.48.09
February	16.59.25R	June	16.32.19	October	17.01.03
March	16.53.42	July	16.32.17D	November	17.13.43
April	16.45.21	August	16.37.51	December	17.23.23

2021

January	17.28.04	May	17.05.08	September	17.15.39
February	17.27.09R	June	17.00.03	October	17.28.32
March	17.21.30	July	16.59.53D	November	17.41.13
April	17.13.13	August	17.05.24	December	17.50.57

2022

January	17.55.43	May	17.32.56	September	17.43.09
February	17.54.54R	June	17.27.47	October	17.56.00
March	17.49.18	July	17.27.34D	November	18.08.43
April	17.41.02	August	17.32.58	December	18.18.31

Appendix 1: Proserpina Ephemeris

Appendix 2. Decan, Term and Degrees Rulers in a Medical Chart

Sign	AR	TA	GE	CA	LE	VI	LI	SC	SA	CP	AQ	PI
1st decan	**Mar**	**Ven**	**Mer**	**Mo**	**Su**	**Pro**	**Chi**	**Plu**	**Jup**	**Sat**	**Ura**	**Nep**
1st term	**Mar**	**Chi**	**Mar**	**Chi**	**Mar**	**Chi**	**Mar**	**Chi**	**Mar**	**Chi**	**Mar**	**Chi**
1	Mar	Chi	Mar	Chi	Mar	Chi	Mar	Chi	Mar	Chi	Mar	Chi
2	Ven	Plu	Ven	Plu	Ven	Plu	Ven	Plu	Ven	Plu	Ven	Plu
3	Mer	Jup	Mer	Jup	Mer	Jup	Mer	Jup	Mer	Jup	Mer	Jup
4	Mo	Sat	Mo	Sat	Mo	Sat	Mo	Sat	Mo	Sat	Mo	Sat
5	Su	Ura	Su	Ura	Su	Ura	Su	Ura	Su	Ura	Su	Ura
2nd term	**Ven**	**Plu**	**Ven**	**Plu**	**Ven**	**Plu**	**Ven**	**Plu**	**Ven**	**Plu**	**Ven**	**Plu**
6	Pro	Nep	Pro	Nep	Pro	Nep	Pro	Nep	Pro	Nep	Pro	Nep
7	Chi	Mar	Chi	Mar	Chi	Mar	Chi	Mar	Chi	Mar	Chi	Mar
8	Plu	Ven	Plu	Ven	Plu	Ven	Plu	Ven	Plu	Ven	Plu	Ven
9	Jup	Mer	Jup	Mer	Jup	Mer	Jup	Mer	Jup	Mer	Jup	Mer
10	Sat	Mo	Sat	Mo	Sat	Mo	Sat	Mo	Sat	Mo	Sat	Mo
2nd decan	**Su**	**Pro**	**Chi**	**Plu**	**Jup**	**Sat**	**Ura**	**Nep**	**Mar**	**Ven**	**Mer**	**Mo**
3rd term	**Mer**	**Jup**	**Mer**	**Jup**	**Mer**	**Jup**	**Mer**	**Jup**	**Mer**	**Jup**	**Mer**	**Jup**
11	Ura	Su	Ura	Su	Ura	Su	Ura	Su	Ura	Su	Ura	Su
12	Nep	Pro	Nep	Pro	Nep	Pro	Nep	Pro	Nep	Pro	Nep	Pro
13	Mar	Chi	Mar	Chi	Mar	Chi	Mar	Chi	Mar	Chi	Mar	Chi
14	Ven	Plu	Ven	Plu	Ven	Plu	Ven	Plu	Ven	Plu	Ven	Plu
15	Mer	Jup	Mer	Jup	Mer	Jup	Mer	Jup	Mer	Jup	Mer	Jup
4th term	**Mo**	**Sat**	**Mo**	**Sat**	**Mo**	**Sat**	**Mo**	**Sat**	**Mo**	**Sat**	**Mo**	**Sat**
16	Mo	Sat	Mo	Sat	Mo	Sat	Mo	Sat	Mo	Sat	Mo	Sat
17	Su	Ura	Su	Ura	Su	Ura	Su	Ura	Su	Ura	Su	Ura
18	Pro	Nep	Pro	Nep	Pro	Nep	Pro	Nep	Pro	Nep	Pro	Nep
19	Chi	Mar	Chi	Mar	Chi	Mar	Chi	Mar	Chi	Mar	Chi	Mar
20	Plu	Ven	Plu	Ven	Plu	Ven	Plu	Ven	Plu	Ven	Plu	Ven
3rd decan	**Jup**	**Sat**	**Ura**	**Nep**	**Mar**	**Ven**	**Mer**	**Mo**	**Su**	**Pro**	**Chi**	**Plu**
5th term	**Su**	**Ura**	**Su**	**Ura**	**Su**	**Ura**	**Su**	**Ura**	**Su**	**Ura**	**Su**	**Ura**
21	Jup	Mer	Jup	Mer	Jup	Mer	Jup	Mer	Jup	Mer	Jup	Mer

22	Sat	Mo	Sat	Mo	Sat	Mo	Sat	Mo	Sat	Mo	Sat	Mo
23	Ura	Su	Ura	Su	Ura	Su	Ura	Su	Ura	Su	Ura	Su
24	Nep	Pro	Nep	Pro	Nep	Pro	Nep	Pro	Nep	Pro	Nep	Pro
25	Mar	Chi	Mar	Chi	Mar	Chi	Mar	Chi	Mar	Chi	Mar	Chi
6th term	**Pro**	**Nep**	**Pro**	**Nep**	**Pro**	**Nep**	**Pro**	**Nep**	**Pro**	**Nep**	**Pro**	**Nep**
26	Ven	Plu	Ven	Plu	Ven	Plu	Ven	Plu	Ven	Plu	Ven	Plu
27	Mer	Jup	Mer	Jup	Mer	Jup	Mer	Jup	Mer	Jup	Mer	Jup
28	Mo	Sat	Mo	Sat	Mo	Sat	Mo	Sat	Mo	Sat	Mo	Sat
29	Su	Ura	Su	Ura	Su	Ura	Su	Ura	Su	Ura	Su	Ura
30	Pro	Nep	Pro	Nep	Pro	Nep	Pro	Nep	Pro	Nep	Pro	Nep

Su: Sun Mo: Moon Mer: Mercury
Ven: Venus Mar: Mars Jup: Jupiter
Sat: Saturn Ura: Uranus Nep: Neptune
Plu: Pluto Chi: Chiron Pro: Proserpina

Appendix 3. Planetary Hours

Hour	Monday L	Monday H	Tuesday L	Tuesday H	Wednesday L	Wednesday H	Thursday L	Thursday H	Friday L	Friday H	Saturday L	Saturday H	Sunday L	Sunday H
1	Mo	Mo	Mar	Plu	Mer	Ura	Jup	Chi	Ven	Nep	Sat	Pro	Su	Su
2	Sat	Pro	Su	Su	Mo	Mo	Mar	Plu	Mer	Ura	Chi	Jup	Ven	Nep
3	Chi	Jup	Ven	Nep	Sat	Pro	Su	Su	Mo	Mo	Plu	Mar	Mer	Ura
4	Plu	Mar	Mer	Ura	Chi	Jup	Ven	Nep	Sat	Pro	Su	Su	Mo	Mo
5	Su	Su	Mo	Mo	Plu	Mar	Mer	Ura	Chi	Jup	Nep	Ven	Sat	Pro
6	Nep	Ven	Sat	Pro	Su	Su	Mo	Mo	Plu	Mar	Ura	Mer	Chi	Jup
7	Ura	Nep	Chi	Jup	Nep	Ven	Sat	Pro	Su	Su	Mo	Mo	Plu	Mar
8	Mo	Mo	Plu	Mar	Ura	Mer	Chi	Jup	Nep	Ven	Pro	Sat	Su	Su
9	Pro	Sat	Su	Su	Mo	Mo	Plu	Mar	Ura	Mer	Jup	Chi	Nep	Ven
10	Jup	Chi	Nep	Ven	Pro	Sat	Su	Su	Mo	Mo	Mar	Plu	Ura	Mer
11	Mar	Plu	Ura	Mer	Jup	Chi	Nep	Ven	Pro	Sat	Su	Su	Mo	Mo
12	Su	Su	Mo	Mo	Mar	Plu	Ura	Mer	Chi	Jup	Ven	Nep	Pro	Sat
13	Ven	Nep	Pro	Sat	Su	Su	Mo	Mo	Mar	Plu	Mer	Ura	Jup	Chi
14	Mer	Ura	Jup	Chi	Ven	Nep	Pro	Sat	Su	Su	Mo	Mo	Mar	Plu
15	Mo	Mo	Mar	Plu	Mer	Ura	Jup	Chi	Ven	Nep	Sat	Pro	Su	Su
16	Sat	Pro	Su	Su	Mo	Mo	Mar	Plu	Mer	Ura	Chi	Jup	Ven	Nep
17	Chi	Jup	Ven	Nep	Sat	Pro	Su	Su	Mo	Mo	Plu	Mar	Mer	Ura
18	Plu	Mar	Mer	Ura	Chi	Jup	Ven	Nep	Sat	Pro	Su	Su	Mo	Mo
19	Su	Su	Mo	Mo	Plu	Mar	Mer	Ura	Chi	Jup	Nep	Ven	Sat	Pro
20	Nep	Ven	Sat	Pro	Su	Su	Mo	Mo	Plu	Mar	Ura	Mer	Chi	Jup
21	Ura	Nep	Chi	Jup	Nep	Ven	Sat	Pro	Su	Su	Mo	Mo	Plu	Mar
22	Mo	Mo	Plu	Mar	Ura	Mer	Chi	Jup	Nep	Ven	Pro	Sat	Su	Su
23	Pro	Sat	Su	Su	Mo	Mo	Plu	Mar	Ura	Mer	Jup	Chi	Nep	Ven
24	Jup	Chi	Nep	Ven	Pro	Sat	Su	Su	Mo	Mo	Mar	Plu	Ura	Mer

Su: Sun
Mo: Moon
Mer: Mercury
Ven: Venus
Mar: Mars
Jup: Jupiter
Sat: Saturn
Ura: Uranus
Nep: Neptune
Plu: Pluto
Chi: Chiron
Pro: Proserpina
L: lower week
H: higher week

Bibliography

Gettings, Fred. *The Arkana Dictionary of Astrology*. London, 1990.

Globa, Pavel. Medical Astrology, lecture. Moscow, 1986.

Globa, Pavel. *Lunnaya Astrologia* (Lunar Astrology). Moscow, 1996.

Phillipova, M.V. *Medicinskaya Astrologia* (Medical Astrology). Moscow, 1993.

Podolsky, Igor. Medical Astrology, lecture. Moscow, 1993.

Zyurnyaeva, Tamara. *Kak Zhit*. Minsk, Belorussia, 1998.

www.ingramcontent.com/pod-product-compliance
Lightning Source LLC
Chambersburg PA
CBHW050501110426
42742CB00018B/3333